Slow Cooker Low Carb

250 Low Carb, Healthy, Delicious, Easy Recipes

Cooking and Recipes for Weight Loss

5th Edition

By

Arianna Brooks

Arianna Brooks

© Copyright 2015-2018 - All rights reserved.

In no way is it legal to reproduce, duplicate, or transmit any part of this document in either electronic means or in printed format. Recording of this publication is strictly prohibited, and any storage of this document is not allowed unless with written permission from the publisher. All rights reserved.

The information provided herein is stated to be truthful and consistent, in that any liability, in terms of inattention or otherwise, by any usage or abuse of any policies, processes, or directions contained within, is the solitary and utter responsibility of the recipient reader. Under no circumstances will any legal responsibility or blame be held against the publisher for any reparation, damages, or monetary loss due to the information herein, either directly or indirectly.

Respective authors own all copyrights not held by the publisher.

Legal Notice:

This eBook is copyright protected. This is only for personal use. You cannot amend, distribute, sell, use, quote or paraphrase any part or the content within this eBook without the consent of the author or copyright owner. Legal action will be pursued if this is breached.

Disclaimer Notice:

Please note the information contained within this document is for educational and entertainment purposes only. Every attempt has been made to provide accurate, up to date, reliable, and complete information. No warranties of any kind

Arianna Brooks

are expressed or implied. Readers acknowledge that the author is not engaging in the rendering of legal, financial, medical or professional advice.

By reading this document, the reader agrees that under no circumstances are we responsible for any losses, direct or indirect, which are incurred as a result of the use of information contained within this document, including, but not limited to, errors, omissions, or inaccuracies.

Table of Contents

Introduction 19

Chapter One: Benefits of following a Low-Carb Diet 21

    They kill your appetite... 22

    They help lose weight 22

    Your energy levels increase 23

    You won't count calories 24

    They help you eat out without awkwardness 24

    Reduced blood sugar levels and facilitate improvement in type 2 diabetes...25

    They help to treat metabolic syndrome 26

    They can improve the LDL cholesterol pattern 27

    They are therapeutic for several brain disorders................27

Chapter Two: Benefits of Slow Cookers 29

    Saving energy 29

    Preserves nutrients... 29

    Cleaning..31

    Eliminates Harmful Microorganisms 32

    What is a low-carb diet?..33

    Slow Cooker Tips and Safety....................................33

Chapter Three - Breakfast 37

Chile, Cheese, and Scrambled Egg Grits 37

Hash brown, Spinach and Ham Casserole 39

Overnight Breakfast Casserole 40

Spinach and Mozzarella Frittata 42

Cream Cheese Easy Egg Bake 44

Savory Breakfast Muffins 45

Spanish Potato Omelet 47

Zucchini Banana Bread with Chocolate Chips 49

Egg and Broccoli Casserole 51

Mexican Breakfast Casserole 52

Italian Beef Sandwiches 53

Slow Cooked Breakfast Pizza 55

Breakfast Casserole 56

Burrito 57

Mushroom and Basil Egg Pie 58

Cauliflower Hash Browns Casserole 59

Egg & Sausage Breakfast Casserole 60

Frittata w/ Roasted Red Pepper, Artichoke Hearts, & Feta 61

Egg, Bacon and Hash Brown Casserole 63

Breakfast Meatloaf 64

Slow Cooker Bacon, Egg & Hash Brown Casserole 66

Slow Cooker Frittata with Artichoke Hearts, Roasted Red Pepper, and Feta 68

Slow Cooker Kale Bacon Breakfast Casserole 70

Breakfast Casserole with Cheese and Sausage (Gluten free) 72

Slow Cooker Frittata with Kale, Roasted Red Pepper, and Feta 74

Greek Eggs Breakfast Casserole 76

Slow Cooker Veggie Omelet 78

Chapter Four - Main Course – Beef 81

Layered Brisket Dinner with Tangy Mustard Sauce 81

Boeuf Bourguignon with Spiralized Vegetables 83

Slow Cooker Picadillo 85

Beef Curry 87

Pepperoni Pizza Chili 88

Crockpot Bolognese 89

Slow Cooked Beef with Carrots and Cabbage 91

Slow Cooker Chipotle Beef Barbacoa 93

Hungarian Beef Goulash 95

Slow-Cooker Braised Beef with Carrots & Turnips 97

Fireside Beef Stew 99

Slow-Cooked Brisket in Onion Gravy 101

French Country Beef Stew 104

Fragrant Shredded Beef Stew 106

Coffee-Braised Pot Roast with Caramelized Onions 108

Texas Beef and Beans 110

Slow Cooker Ham and Egg Casserole 111

Low Carb Chili 113

Simple Pepper Steak 115

Easy Italian Steak 117

Beer-braised Short Ribs 118

Barbecue Brisket 119

Beef Roast with Apples 120

Sour Cream Pot Roast 121

Mexican Steak Stew 122

Beef with Eggplant 123

Beef Osso Buco 124

Mexican Beef 126

Beef Pot Roast with Mushrooms 128

Spicy Braised Beef 129

Puerto Rican Beef Encebollado 130

Traditional Ropa Vieja 131

Hearty Beef Stew 133

Stuffed Peppers 135

Kicking Chili 136

Beef Rags 138

Swiss Steak 140

Coffee Brisket 141

Beef and Beans 142

Beef Stroganoff 143

Autumn Oxtail Stew 145

Corned Beef & Cabbage 147

Tri-Tip Tacos 148

Ropa Vieja Variation 150

Korean Beef Tacos 151

Beef Machaca 153

Italian Beef 154

Beef Ragu 155

Shredded Asian Beef 156

Thai Curry Ground Beef 157

Chapter Five - Main Course - Pork and Lamb......... 159

Pork Stroganoff 159

Pork Paprikash..161

Italian Pork Tenderloin 163

North African Lamb Shanks 164

Moroccan Lamb Shoulders... 166

Lamb Curry 168

Spanish Lamb with Sherry, Honey & Peppers 170

Slow-Cooker Braised Pork with Salsa 172

Sage-Scented Pork Chops 174

Mushroom-Sauced Pork Chops..176

Slow-Cooker Baby Back Ribs... 178

Slow-Cooker Char Siu Pork 180

Fennel & Pork Stew.. 182

Chinese Pork & Vegetable Hot Pot 184

Hoisin Pork in Lettuce cups 186

Mushroom and Pork Chops... 187

Oriental Pork Roast 188

Leg of Lamb 189

Apple and Cranberry Pork Roast....................................... 190

Pork Chops in Beer 191

Lamb Stew 192

Lamb Paprikash 193

Maple Pork Ribs 194

Pork Stuffed Peppers 195

Tender and Tangy Pork Brisket 196

Pork Adobado 197

Pizza Meatloaf 199

Lamb Chops 201

Pork Tenderloin 202

Roasted Pork 203

Simple Pork Chops 205

Camitas 206

Paprika Pork Tenderloin 208

Cochinita Pibil 209

Lamb Shanks w/ Cannellini Beans 211

Amazing Slow Cooked Pork Tenderloin 213

Pork with Beans & Greens 214

Diet Cola Pot Roast 216

Barbecue Pulled Pot Roast 217

Cuban-Style Pot Roast 219

Balsamic Bacon Meatloaf Barbecue 221

Chapter Six - Main Course - Chicken and Turkey ... 223

Slow Cooked Tahini Chicken Thighs 223

Cherry Tomato Chicken Cacciatore 224

Chicken Lo Mein 225

Creamy Sundried Tomato Chicken 227

Slow Cooker Chicken Creole 229

Slow Cooker Jerk Chicken 231

Slow Cooker Chicken Fajitas 233

Slow Cooker Balsamic Chicken 236

Buffalo Chicken Salads 239

Rosemary Chicken 241

Slow-Cooker Vietnamese Pulled Chicken 243

Savory Barbecue Chicken 245

Shredded Chicken Master Recipe 246

Slow-Cooker Chicken Parmesan Meatballs 248

Wine & Tomato Braised Chicken 250

Chicken and Pepperoni 252

Barbecue Pulled Chicken 254

Asian Style Slow Cooked Chicken Wings 256

Italian Chicken 258

Chicken in Wine Sauce 259

Thai Chicken 260

Curried Chicken with Tomatoes 261

Oriental Ginger Chicken 262

Stuffed Chicken Breast 263

Roast Turkey Breast 264

Chicken Parmesan 265

Olive Oil and Rosemary Chicken 266

Cheesy Chicken 267

Salsa Chicken 268

Neufchatel Chicken 269

Lemon Chicken 270

Vegetable and Herbed Chicken Stew 271

Thai Green Chicken Curry 272

Gourmet Chicken 273

Orange Chicken 274

Indian Butter Chicken 275

Mediterranean Roast Turkey 277

Asian Braised Turkey with Vegetables 278

Jamaican Jerk Chicken 280

Spicy Chicken Drumsticks 281

Greek-Style Stuffed Chicken Breasts 282

Buffalo Chicken 284

Butter Chicken Special 285

Pollo Pibil 287

Chicken Barbacoa 289

Eggplant Turkey Bolognese 290

Roasted Sticky Chicken 291

Marinara Chicken & Veggies 292

Mustard Honey Turkey Stew 293

Chicken Gyros 294

Chicken Marsala 296

Slow Cooker Turkey Breast with Gravy 298

Crockpot Turkey Breast 300

Chapter Seven - Soups 303

Green Eggs & Ham Soup 303

Chicken-Corn Tortilla Soup 305

Rainbow Vegetable Soup 307

Slow-Cooker Hot & Sour Soup 308

Barbecue Meatball Soup 310

Inestrone Soup with Pork 312

Curried Butternut Squash Soup 314

Asparagus & Sorrel Bisque 315

Creamy Chicken Noodle Soup 317

Ginger-Chicken Noodle Soup 319

Roasted Tomato and Vegetable Soup 321

Low-Carb Pumpkin and Coconut Soup 323

Pumpkin Soup 324

Tomato Soup 325

Cauliflower Soup 326

Broccoli Soup 327

Mexican Chicken Chowder 328

Summer Vegetable Soup 329

California-Style Seafood Soup 330

Spicy Chicken Soup 332

Moqueca de Camaroes (Brazilian Shrimp Soup) 333

Pizza Soup 334

Cheese Burger Soup 335

Spicy Thai Chicken Soup 337

Turkey Soup 339

Onion Soup 341

Chicken Fajita Soup 342

Italian Sausage and Lentil Soup 343

Rueben Soup 345

Mulligatawny Soup 346

Spinach, Tomato, Vegetable Soup 348

Vegetable Soup 349

Zucchini Soup 350

Minestrone Veggie Soup 351

Cream of Asparagus Soup 353

Chicken Parmesan Soup 354

Italian Low Carb Wedding Soup 355

Hot Chicken Cabbage Soup 357

Split Pea & Ham Soup 358

Chapter Eight – Dips, Stews, Snacks & Sausages ... 359

Lamb Ropa Vieja (Cuban Lamb Stew) 359

Hearty Chicken Stew 361

Gruyere – Bacon Dip 363

Hot Cheesy Roasted Brussels Sprout Dip 365

Grain Free Granola 366

Cranberry-Citrus Meatballs 368

Italian Cocktail Meatballs 370

Apricot-Honey Mustard Sausage Bites 371

Slow-Cooker Buffalo Chicken Dip 372

Cheese Fondue with Fennel & Tomatoes 374

Bourbon-Glazed Cocktail Sausages 376

Slow-Cooker Chicken Enchilada Dip 377

Middle Eastern Lamb Stew 379

Low Carb Chipotle Cauliflower Cheese 381

Slow Cooker Lamb with Thyme 383

Mustard Cocktail Sausages 384

Low Carb Buffalo Almonds 385

Low Carb BBQ Party Sausages 386

Chapter Nine - Desserts 387

Pumpkin Pie Pudding 387

Chocolate Truffle Crème Brulee 388

Mocha Pudding Cake 390

Slow Cooker Baby Bok Choy Brownies 392

Blueberry Lemon Custard Cake 394

Healthy Chocolate Muffins 396

Slow-Cooker Chai Apple Butter 398

Slow Cooker Low Carb Maple Custard 400

Slow Cooker Low Carb Mint Chocolate Cake 402

Low Carb Chocolate Fondue 404

Slow Cooker Dark Chocolate Cake 405

Slow Cooker Raspberry Cream Cheese Cake 407

Flan 409

Pumpkin Pie Custard 410

Carrot Pudding 411

Dark Chocolate Cake.. 412

Pumpkin Spice Cake 413

Carrot Cake with Cream Cheese 414

Gingerbread 416

Sugar-Free Molten Lava Chocolate Cake 418

Pumpkin Pie Bars (Sugar-Free) 420

Dairy and Refined Sugar-Free Fudge................................ 422

Lemon Poke Cake 423

Conclusion 427

Introduction

Thank you for purchasing my latest cookbook, *"Slow Cooker: Low Carb: 250 Low Carb, Healthy, Delicious, Easy Recipes: Cooking and Recipes for Weight Loss"*. I really hope you enjoy the following Low Carb meals.

This book contains recipes on how to prepare delicious and healthy meals using your slow cooker that are low carb and I hope assist you in eating healthier and achieving your weight loss goals.

I've found losing weight, maintaining a healthy figure, and keeping fit have all become so much easier when you have a slow cooker in your kitchen. No matter how busy your daily schedule is, you can still enjoy healthy meals because with a slow cooker, all you have to do is throw together the ingredients in the pot, put it on the right settings, and leave it alone while you go about your day.

The recipes in this book will help you to lose weight and live a healthier lifestyle by enjoying a low carb diet that is rich in vitamins, minerals, and essential nutrients. Use your slow cooker to its full advantage by letting it do all the cooking for you as you go about your daily schedule.

In this book, you will find slow cooker breakfast recipes, beef, pork, lamb, chicken, and turkey main course recipes, soup recipes, and dessert recipes.

Let this be an opportunity for you to make your health a top priority. Nourish yourself with hot, healthy, and delicious foods and experience looking and feeling great.

Thanks again for purchasing this book, I hope you enjoy it!

Arianna Brooks

Chapter One: Benefits of following a Low-Carb Diet

Do you remember the time when the low-carb diet was getting all the attention in the media in the 1990s? A lot of people had passed off the low-carb diet as just another diet fad, and I don't blame them. After all, how could you believe that a diet that requires you to reduce your carbohydrate intake can be healthy at all? I mean sure, you could end up losing weight, but how is it going to be truly healthy for anyone? Some were even concerned about whether the low-carb diet could increase the risk of developing cardiovascular disease.

A lot of time has passed since then, and scientists all over the world have conducted extensive research about the low-carb diet. The best part about a low-carb diet is that it's not only proven to be healthy, but it also helps you lose weight, without counting calories. How many diets offer you the luxury of not having to constantly watch your calories? I bet none of them.

Low-carb diets may have been controversial in the past, but today, they are the most trusted and go-to diets for anyone who wants to lose weight and maintain it in a much healthier fashion. Since 2002, there have been over 20 studies conducted on low-carb diets, all of which have concluded that such diets are superior to other diets.

Let's talk about the benefits of the ketogenic diet and low-carb diet.

They kill your appetite

Yes, but in a good way! What's the one thing that stops people from following their diet plans? Hunger. It can be considered as the biggest side effect of dieting. Don't you feel ravenously hungry, especially when you are in the midst of a diet plan? For some reason, it feels like your appetite has doubled, and you can't stop yourself from reaching for an extra serving of meat. This feeling is the primary reason why people start feeling miserable about themselves and eventually lose the motivation to stick to their diets. This is why low-carb diets work. The best thing about a low-carb diet is that it naturally reduces your appetite. Several studies have shown that individuals who are placed on low-carb diets end up feeling less hungry. When people start cutting down on carbs while increasing their protein and fat intake, they feel fuller most of the time. This helps to maintain portion control without having to put in extra efforts to exercise any self-control over yourself – simply because you aren't hungry anymore.

They help lose weight

Cutting down carbs is the easiest and the most effective way to lose that excess weight. Several studies have shown that individuals who are on low-carb diets end up losing a lot of water weight in the first few weeks, which causes drastic weight loss. Low-carb diets are known to reduce a person's insulin levels while causing the kidneys to shed excess sodium, resulting in rapid weight loss in the first couple of weeks. A lot of dieters are pleasantly surprised when they end up losing a significant amount of weight within such a short duration, and this motivates them further to stick to the diet.

Studies that compared low-fat and low-carb diets have shown that people who follow a low-carb diet can lose up to three times as much weight without feeling hungry. That being said, low-carb diets work particularly well for the first six months, but later on, the weight starts coming back. This happens because people tend to go back to their old dietary habits once they have achieved their desired weight loss, and so they start piling up calories again. Thus, if you wish to maintain the weight loss, make sure that you make this diet a part of your lifestyle.

Your energy levels increase

Have you noticed your blood sugar levels taking a roller-coaster ride when you are on carb-overdrive? One minute, your mood is up, but the next minute, it's down in the dumps. Take the post-lunch afternoon crash as an example. A big slice of pizza, or a bowl of leftover cheesy pasta from last night, can seem extremely satisfying and convenient at the moment, but soon, this carbo-loading can set you up for a major fall a couple of hours down the line. This can take a serious toll on your energy levels, both physical and mental; in fact, in the worst case, this can also create anxiety in people.

When it comes to low-carb diets, you will not face any of these problems. Cutting down carbohydrates from the diet helps you enter a state of ketosis, causing your blood sugar levels to stabilize. This is exactly what prevents the proverbial roller coaster effect, allowing you to control your emotions effectively. If you continue this diet for a week or two, you will feel more in tune with yourself and have more energy to get through the day.

You won't count calories

Oh, I love this part!! Not having to count calories has to be the highlight of this diet. There are so many diets that focus on a drastic reduction in calories, assuming that fewer calories could equal weight loss. Of course, this works for a few days; you may even start losing weight with this technique, but along with the weight, you may also start losing your skin, hair, and overall health. Such fad diets are only good if you are looking for short-term weight loss. However, it's neither a sustainable nor a healthy way to live. Even if you stick to your daily calorie limits, you will deny yourself the most essential nutrients your body actually needs.

Back to my favorite part about the low-carb diet, you don't have to watch what you put in your mouth. Low-carb diets are not about how many calories you are ingesting but more about what you are consuming. Certainly, a thing like too many calories exists, but not all of them are created equally. For example, 1000 calories from carb-rich processed foods are different from the 1000 calories you get from eating protein and fat.

They help you eat out without awkwardness

Yay! No more worrying about whether the menu has what your diet approves of when you are eating out. One of the things I found would make my life difficult while following other diets is that I could not go on family dinners or parties anymore. The menu served at these places would consist of everything that was forbidden. Needless to say, I would give up these diets sooner than I thought.

Low-carb diets are totally different. You can have all the meat and fish in the world you want. You can also dig into salmon and a whole load of butter with some veggies on the side. How cool is that? You might need to ask the chef to add an extra ingredient or two, but any good restaurant would be happy to accommodate your request. The very fact that you can go out for social gatherings and parties or eat at restaurants while still able to effortlessly maintain your diet can put you at peace.

Reduced blood sugar levels and facilitate improvement in type 2 diabetes

When you eat carbs, your body breaks them down into simple sugars in your digestive tract. It is from here that they enter your bloodstream and start elevating your blood sugar levels. At worst, they can wreak havoc in the body, and you may need immediate medical attention to bring your blood sugar levels down. High blood sugar levels are extremely toxic for the body. The body responds to a spike in blood sugar levels with a hormone called insulin, which helps to transmit glucose in the cells and later helps burn or store it.

In healthier individuals, this type of instant insulin rise tends to reduce blood sugar spikes to save them from harm. However, a lot of people have a faulty system, and they suffer from what they call "insulin resistance," such that their bodies may end up reacting badly to these sugar spikes. This condition can also lead to type 2 diabetes, where a person's body fails to release enough insulin to decrease the blood sugar levels of an individual after a meal. There is still a simple solution to this problem – cutting down carbohydrates. According to a particular study conducted among type 2 diabetics, 95.2% of them were able to eliminate or reduce their glucose-lowering medicines just within a span of six months.

They help to treat metabolic syndrome

The metabolic syndrome is actually a serious medical condition that is linked to the risk of developing heart diseases and diabetes.

This medical condition is a collection of various symptoms:

- Low HDL levels
- Elevated blood pressure
- Abdominal obesity
- Elevated fasting blood sugar levels
- High triglycerides

A person suffering from metabolic syndrome might be suffering from all or most of the above symptoms. The good news is that all these symptoms can be improved by going on a low-carb diet. Carbohydrates are the primary stimulus for insulin; hence, reducing a person's carbohydrate intake can be impactful in restoring insulin responses. One should remember that it's about reducing the carbohydrate intake, not the fat intake.

As more and more people are reportedly becoming obese, metabolic syndrome is becoming a rather pervasive problem all across the world. Researchers emphasize that one can also cure metabolic syndrome through lifestyle changes. A low-carb diet is a classic demonstration of a lifestyle change doesn't just treat but also possibly cures metabolic syndrome.

They can improve the LDL cholesterol pattern

Low-density lipoprotein (LDL) is often termed as bad cholesterol when, in reality, it's just a protein. Research has shown that people who have increased LDL levels are much more likely to experience heart attacks than those with lower LDL levels. However, several scientists have now discovered that it's not the amount of LDL in the body but the type of LDL that really matters. Not all LDLs are created equal. Going by the same principle, even the size of particles is important. Research has also shown that people who have mostly tiny particles of LDL cholesterol in their bodies are at a high risk of developing heart diseases, whereas those who have large particles of LDL in their bodies are less likely to develop heart disease.

It has also become evident that low-carb diets have the ability to transform small LDL particles into large ones while decreasing the number of LDL particles floating around a person's bloodstream. If you are suffering from heart diseases, you need to start reducing your carbohydrate intake while loading up on healthy fats and proteins in your diet. Fresh fruits, vegetables, and exercise can also significantly reduce the impact of such a disease.

They are therapeutic for several brain disorders

We have read about how important glucose is for the brain to function properly, and a large part of it is true! There's a certain part of the brain that can only burn glucose, and that is one reason why the liver produces glucose from proteins without you having to eat any carbs at all. Nevertheless, a large part of the brain is also capable of burning ketones, which are formed when a person's carbohydrate consumption is low or when he or she is starving. This is the exact mechanism behind low-carb diets, which are being used to treat epilepsy in children for decades. Children who suffer from epilepsy and don't respond to drug treatment are put on a low-carb diet as a part of the treatment.

In several cases, the low-carb diet alone has cured these children of epilepsy. In one study, children who were placed on low-carb diets had a more than 50% reduction in seizures, while 16% had turned seizure-free. Very low-carb diets are even being studied for brain disorders, such as Parkinson's disease and Alzheimer's disease.

Chapter Two: Benefits of Slow Cookers

Slow cooking has several advantages, such as saving time and energy, preserving the nutrients in food, and eliminating all harmful microorganisms that might be present in food. Let us look at all the different benefits of slow cooking.

Saving energy

Slow cooking is a wonderful cooking technique. When you use this method of cooking, you reduce the time spent in the kitchen considerably. You no longer have to slave away in the kitchen. You merely toss all the ingredients in a pot and wait for the food to cook. If you want to enjoy home-cooked meals but don't like the idea of spending hours in the kitchen, then slow cooking is the method for you. While your meal cooks itself, you can do other chores at home. A slow cooker is a wonderful kitchen appliance, and once you use it, you will certainly fall in love with it.

Preserves nutrients

Cooking with a slow cooker will help ensure that heat is spread evenly and that food is cooked uniformly. A slow cooker consists of a lidded round cooking pot that is usually made of either glazed ceramic or porcelain. The cooking pot is surrounded by metal that houses the heating element. The condensed vapor collects in the groove of the inner pot and creates a low-pressure atmosphere that cooks the food. A slow cooker is different from a regular pressure cooker, and unlike the latter, it doesn't present the danger of abruptly releasing pressure. The heat from the heating element is transferred to the cooking pot, and it helps cook the food. This technique of cooking ensures that all the nutrients in the food, such as various minerals and vitamins, will stay intact and won't dissipate. Steam will surround the food, and this means that the food wouldn't get oxidized by air or exposure to heat. Therefore, fresh green foods will retain their color, even after being cooked.

A slow cooker has a unique cooking mechanism where the food stays fully sealed. No steam or any smells will spread throughout your home or your kitchen. This makes for a clean and extremely convenient cooking appliance. A slow cooker is best suited for cooking flavorful meals that retain all their nutrients. Owing to the cooking cycles that are controlled by the heat settings, all the meals are cooked in a consistent manner.

The food that is cooked in a slow cooker is cooked in a fully sealed container. This means that all the nutrients and flavors in the ingredients are trapped within the container. The water content and fresh juices within all the ingredients will remain in the cooking pot and will not dissipate.

You can cook any cut of meat to perfection using this appliance. Even if you use a tough cut of meat or any of the cheaper cuts, you will still be able to cook it to perfection. In fact, this is the best appliance to braise or tenderize meats. You can cook the meat perfectly so that it is falling off the bone. For instance, you make hearty stews using cheap cuts of meat. Not only will you be able to feast on a delicious meal, but it will be lighter on your pocket as well.

Another important feature of this appliance is that all meals will be cooked consistently. This is possible because of the heating mechanism that ensures that similar foods are cooked in a similar manner and also due to the even distribution of heat while cooking. When you cook food at a constant temperature for a prolonged period, the results will be consistent as well.

Cleaning

Conventional cookers have an image of these spitting and steaming monstrous pots that keep making rattling noises that can scare even an adult. Even if you enjoy cooking, the thought of cleaning up afterwards can make you feel otherwise. The thought of spending an hour or two in the kitchen, cleaning all the pots and pans, will prevent you from cooking. If you enjoy cooking but don't like cleaning up afterwards, then the slow cooker is the perfect kitchen appliance for you. All that you need to clean is a single pot, and that's about it. The slow cooker is fully sealed, and no steam will escape into the immediate environment. Therefore, you don't have to worry about any smells spreading in your kitchen or your home. As mentioned earlier, it will help trap all the flavors of the food within the container. A slow cooker will help you to cook food without heating up the surroundings, and this will be well appreciated during summer time by reducing the electricity required for heating and cooling the food. The slow cooker certainly helps you keep your kitchen clean. There won't be any messy spills or splashes, and you don't have to clean up food that boils over. Everything is perfectly sealed and trapped within the inner pot. It is a kitchen friendly appliance that requires minimal cleaning. It is a multipurpose appliance, and it will help you get rid of the clutter in your kitchen.

Arianna Brooks

Eliminates Harmful Microorganisms

When food is cooked at a temperature that is above the boiling point of water, then this will help kill all the harmful microorganisms that might be present in the ingredients like bacteria and viruses. Slow cooking is a good way to sterilize your food. Rice, wheat, corn, and even beans tend to carry different fungal poisons referred to as aflatoxins. These aflatoxins are produced by different species of fungi due to humid conditions and improper storage. In addition, these are responsible for triggering a range of potent illnesses, such as liver cancer, and might also play a role in hosting other triggers of cancer. Well, you don't have to worry about these toxins because a low-carb diet effectively eliminates all forms of carbs. Just heating the food to the boiling point of water does not necessarily destroy these harmful toxins. Cooking it at that temperature really helps. Kidney beans are a very common ingredient and are mostly used in cooking chili. Well, these kidney beans have a particular toxin that's present in them, and the only way this can be destroyed is by cooking the beans at a really high temperature for at least 10 minutes. Certain meats like chicken and pork need to be cooked thoroughly to kill certain harmful microorganisms present in them. When you cook meat in a slow cooker, all the time it takes to cook the meat automatically ensures that there are no harmful microorganisms left behind.

The slow cooker also frees up all the space in your oven and stovetop for other purposes. In fact, it is a good idea to cook meals in a slow cooker for large gatherings. You can make a pot of delicious and nutritious soup using your slow cooker. Slow cookers also utilize less energy than a conventional electric oven. Moreover, when you cook food at a low temperature, the chances of burning the food or scorching it also tends to reduce. Apart from all these, a slow cooker is quite portable and travel-friendly. You simply need to plug it in at your office or at the party, and you can enjoy hot food instantly.

Well, a slow cooker is a marvelous kitchen appliance. All that you need is one appliance to cook your meals in. Go through the various recipes given in this book to cook delicious and nutritious meals in no time.

What is a low-carb diet?

Like the name suggests, this is a diet that is rich in proteins and dietary fats but limits the consumption of carbs. If you want to improve your overall health by making a couple of simple changes to your diet, then a low-carb diet would be the perfect fit for you. The major source of energy will be proteins and food rich in dietary fats.

Slow Cooker Tips and Safety

Do you want to be able to whip up tasty food without having to spend hours in the kitchen? Well then the Instant Pot is the right appliance for you. The slow cooker is quite handy and very simple to use. It will not only save you time and effort, but it can also improve your overall health. A slow cooker makes use of pressurized steam to help you cook meals, and this method helps to seal most of the nutrients in food.

If you are hesitant about trying a slow cooker and cooking while you are away throughout the day, then you can consider cooking during alternate hours when you are at home. You simply need to toss all the ingredients into this appliance and then wait for it to work its magic. In the meantime, you can take a quick nap, shop for groceries, or even get some household chores done. You can even cook in batches and freeze the leftovers. So during the week, you merely need to heat up the food, and voila – you can enjoy a nutritious meal quickly!

Here are some basic tips and safety rules that you must keep in mind while using a slow cooker.

If you are looking for a means to quickly clean the slow cooker, then make sure that you rub the inside pot of the stoneware with some oil or nonstick cooking spray before you use it. Alternatively, you can use slow cooker liners to ease up this process. Instead of cleaning a variety of pots and pans, you only need to clean one slow cooker, and that's it.

Before you use any frozen meat or other frozen produce, you need to thaw it before tossing it into the slow cooker. If you don't thaw the meat, then it will not cook evenly. If you want your meat to cook evenly, then don't forget to thaw it once you remove it from the refrigerator.

You must fill the slow cooker to no more than 2/3 of its capacity and no less than ½ of its capacity. If you cook too little or too much, then it will affect the cooking time, the quality of the food, and also the safety.

Vegetables take a while longer to cook than poultry or meat. So you need to place the vegetables first in the slow cooker, then place the meat on top of the vegetables, and top it all off with some water, broth, or any sauce that you are using.

You can use a slow cooker to reduce any liquids like broth. You can simmer the liquid in the slow cooker until it is of the desired consistency. Liquids don't boil away in a slow cooker, so you don't have to worry about burning the cooking pot.

If you remove the lid, then it will slow down the cooking process. So you need to make sure that the lid stays on, unless the recipe suggests otherwise. Every time you remove the lid, you lose about 15 to 20 minutes of the cooking time. When you remove the lid, the heat that is building up in the pot is released, which is what increases the cooking time.

If you need to use milk, cheese, or cream in a certain recipe, make sure that you add it in the last hour. You cannot slow cook dairy products for long because they stand the risk of curdling.

Arianna Brooks

Chapter Three - Breakfast

Chile, Cheese, and Scrambled Egg Grits

Makes: 4 servings

Carbs per serving: 15 grams

Ingredients:

- 2 ¼ cups chicken broth or vegetable broth
- ¼ teaspoon ground cumin
- 6 tablespoons low fat Cheddar cheese, shredded
- 1 clove garlic, minced
- Salt to taste
- ½ cup yellow or white grits
- ½ can (from a 4 ounces can) diced green chili peppers with a little of the liquid
- 2 eggs
- Nonstick cooking spray

Instructions:

1. Place a disposable liner on the bottom of the slow cooker pot. Spray cooking spray over the liner.
2. Add broth, cumin, grits, cheese, garlic, salt to taste and green chili along with a little of the canned liquid into a bowl and stir until well combined. Pour into the pot.
3. Cover the pot and cook on low for 6-8 hours or on high for 3 to 4 hours. Stir once after 3 hours. When the timer goes off, switch off the cooker.
4. Add eggs into a bowl. Add a pinch of salt and beat well. Spoon the egg over the grits.

5. Cover and let it sit for 30 minutes. Stir well.
6. Ladle into bowls and serve.

Hash brown, Spinach and Ham Casserole

Makes: 3 servings

Carbs per serving: 14 grams

Ingredients:

- 5 oz. hash brown potatoes, refrigerated or defrosted if frozen
- 1/8 cup onions, diced
- 5 oz. frozen spinach, defrosted, drained
- 3 egg whites
- 3 eggs
- 2 tablespoons skim milk
- Pepper to taste
- Salt to taste
- ½ green bell pepper, chopped
- 2 oz. frozen spinach, defrosted, drained
- 2 oz. lean ham, boneless, chopped

Instructions:

1. Spray the slow cooker pot with cooking spray.
2. Add hash browns, bell pepper and onion into a bowl and mix well. Transfer into the slow cooker. Press it well on to the bottom of the pot. Sprinkle salt and pepper over it.
3. Add spinach and ham in a bowl and stir. Spread over the hash brown layer. Sprinkle cheese.
4. Add eggs, whites, salt, pepper and milk into a bowl and whisk well. Pour over the spinach layer.
5. Cover the pot and cook on low for 4-6 hours or on high for 2-3 hours.

Arianna Brooks

Overnight Breakfast Casserole

Makes: 5 servings

Carbs per serving: 8.2 grams

Ingredients:

- ¼ pound bulk breakfast sausage, crumbled
- ¼ cup yellow onion, diced
- ½ orange bell pepper, deseeded, diced
- ½ red bell pepper, deseeded, diced
- 3 ounces bacon, chopped
- ½ pound sweet potatoes, peeled, shredded
- 2 teaspoons ghee, softened, to grease
- 2 tablespoons full fat coconut milk
- ¼ cup almond milk
- 8 large eggs, well beaten
- ½ teaspoon dry mustard
- Cracked black pepper to taste
- ½teaspoon sea salt
- 1 green onion, thinly sliced

Instructions:

1. Grease the inside of the slow cooker with ghee.
2. Place a skillet over medium high heat. Add sausage, bacon and onions. Sauté until the sausages are brown and onions are pink. Turn off the heat. Drain the fat remaining in the skillet.
3. Place the sweet potatoes in the cooker. Spread it all over the bottom of the cooker and press it lightly.
4. Add the sausage mixture and bell pepper.

5. Add eggs, almond milk, coconut milk, salt, pepper and mustard into a bowl and whisk well. Pour it over the sausages in the pot.
6. Cover the pot and cook on low for 6 to 8 hours.

Arianna Brooks

Spinach and Mozzarella Frittata

Makes: 12 servings

Carbs per serving: 4 grams

Ingredients:

- 2 tablespoons extra-virgin olive oil
- 2 cups 2% fat mozzarella cheese, divided
- 6 egg whites
- 6 eggs
- ¼ cup 1% milk
- ½ teaspoon white pepper powder
- ½ teaspoon black pepper powder
- Salt to taste
- 2 Roma tomatoes, diced
- 1 cup onion, chopped
- 2 cups packed spinach, shredded, discard stem
- Olive oil or canola oil cooking spray

Instructions:

1. Grease the inside of the slow cooker by spraying with cooking spray.
2. Place a skillet over medium heat. Add oil. When the oil is heated, add onions and sauté until translucent. Transfer into a bowl.
3. Add 1 ½ cups Mozzarella cheese, eggs, egg whites, milk, salt, tomato, spinach, white and black pepper powder into the bowl of onions. Mix until well combined.
4. Spoon into the prepared slow cooker. Sprinkle ½ cup Mozzarella cheese on top.

5. Cover the pot and cook on Low for 1 ½-2 hours or until set. A knitting needle when inserted in the center of the frittata should come out clean.

Arianna Brooks

Cream Cheese Easy Egg Bake

Makes: 8 servings

Carbs per serving: 2 grams

Ingredients:

For egg mixture

- 8 oz. cream cheese
- Salt to taste
- 8 eggs
- 2/3 cup half and half
- Cooking spray

For toppings

- 1 teaspoon-dried herbs of your choice like oregano, basil, etc.
- 2 cups cheddar or Mozzarella cheese, shredded
- 1 teaspoon dried onion
- 1 teaspoon dried minced garlic

Instructions:

1. Grease the inside of the slow cooker by spraying with cooking spray.
2. Add cream cheese, salt, eggs and half and half into a blender and blend until well combined.
3. Pour into the cooker. Sprinkle dried herbs, cheese, onion and garlic.
4. Cover the pot and cook on Low for 4-5 hours or on High for 2- 2 ½ hours.

Savory Breakfast Muffins

Makes: 6 servings

Carbs per serving: 6 grams

Ingredients:

For dry ingredients

- ¼ cup almond meal
- ¼ cup Parmesan cheese, finely grated
- 2 tablespoons nutritional yeast flakes
- ¼ teaspoon spike seasoning (optional)
- ¼ cup raw hemp seeds
- 2 tablespoons flaxseed meal
- ¼ teaspoon gluten free baking powder
- 1/8 teaspoon salt or to taste

For wet ingredients

- 3 eggs, beaten
- 1 green onion, thinly sliced
- ¼ cup low fat cottage cheese

Instructions:

1. Grease 6 muffin molds with some oil or butter. You can also use silicone muffin cups.
2. Combine the dry ingredients in a bowl.
3. Add all the wet ingredients into a large bowl and whisk until well incorporated.
4. Add the mixture of dry ingredients into the bowl of wet ingredients, a little at a time and whisk well each time until the batter is smooth and free from lumps. Spoon into the prepared muffin molds. Fill up to ¾.

5. Place a rack on the bottom of the slow cooker or crumple some aluminum foil and place on the bottom of the cooker. (This need not be done if your cooking pot is ceramic). Place the muffin molds inside the cooker.
6. Cover the pot and cook on high and set the timer for 2-3 hours. Check after 2 hours of cooking. A toothpick when inserted in the center of the muffin should come out clean if the muffins are done. If it is not looking done, then cook for some more time. If you like the top to be dry, then uncover and cook during the last 40-60 minutes of cooking. For medium top, you can place a chopstick on the top of the cooker before closing the lid.
7. Switch off the cooker and remove the lid. Let it cool in the cooker for a while.
8. Run a knife around the edges. Invert onto a plate and serve.
9. Leftovers can be stored in an airtight container in the refrigerator for 6-7 days. Heat in a microwave and serve.

Spanish Potato Omelet

Makes: 4 servings

Carbs per serving: 11 grams

Ingredients:

- ½ pound russet potatoes, peeled, cut into ¾ inch pieces
- ¼ cup onion, chopped
- Black pepper powder to taste
- ¼ cup low fat cheddar cheese, shredded
- 1 tablespoon olive oil
- Salt to taste
- 6 eggs, lightly beaten
- 1 small tomato, chopped
- Nonstick cooking spray

Instructions:

1. Place a disposable liner on the bottom of the slow cooker pot. Spray cooking spray over the liner.
2. Place a skillet over medium heat. Add oil. When the oil is heated, add potatoes and cook until light brown. Stir every 2 minutes.
3. Stir in the onions and sauté until onions are translucent. Stir frequently. Turn off the heat.
4. Spoon the mixture into the pot. Pour beaten eggs into the pot and stir until the potatoes are well coated with the egg.
5. Cover the pot and cook on Low for 2 hours or until done.
6. Run a knife around the edges of the omelet and remove the omelet from the liner.

7. Remove on to a plate. Scatter cheese on top and cover the plate with foil. Let it sit for a few minutes.
8. Slice into 4 wedges. Garnish with tomatoes and serve.

Zucchini Banana Bread with Chocolate Chips

Makes: 8 servings

Carbs per serving: 11 grams

Ingredients:

- 6 tablespoons coconut flour
- ½ teaspoon pure vanilla extract
- 3 teaspoons pure maple syrup
- ¼ teaspoon baking soda
- ½ teaspoon baking powder
- A pinch sea salt
- ¾ teaspoon ground cinnamon
- ½ cup zucchini, finely grated, squeezed of excess moisture
- 3 large eggs, at room temperature
- 1 medium very ripe banana, mashed
- 1 tablespoon coconut oil, melted
- 1/8 teaspoon ground nutmeg
- 2 oz. dark chocolate, chopped into pieces or 2 oz. chocolate chips

Instructions:

1. Grease a bread pan with oil. Line with parchment paper so that some paper is hanging from the sides of the pan.
2. Add oil, eggs, oil, maple syrup, vanilla, nutmeg, cinnamon and banana into a bowl and beat with an electric hand mixer until smooth and creamy.
3. Add coconut flour, baking soda, baking powder and salt. Whisk until well combined. Add zucchini and most of the chocolate chips and stir.

4. Pour the batter into the prepared bread pan. Sprinkle the remaining chocolate chips on top.
5. Place a rack on the bottom of the slow cooker or crumple some aluminum foil and place on the bottom of the cooker. (This need not be done if your cooking pot is ceramic). Place the muffin molds inside the cooker.
6. Cover the pot and cook on High for 2-3 hours. Check after 2 hours of cooking. A toothpick when inserted in the center of the bread should come out clean if the bread is done. If it is not looking done, then cook for some more time. If you like the top to be dry, then uncover and cook during the last 40-60 minutes of cooking. For medium top, you can place a chopstick on the top of the cooker before closing the lid.
7. Switch off the cooker and remove the lid. Let it cool in the cooker for a while.
8. Cool completely. Cut into 8 slices and serve.

Egg and Broccoli Casserole

Makes: 3 servings

Carbs per serving: 12 grams

Ingredients:

- 3/4 cup beaten egg or egg substitute
- 5 oz frozen broccoli, thawed and drained
- 12 oz. cottage cheese
- 1/6 cup flour
- 1/8 cup melted unsalted butter
- 1 1/2 Tbsp. finely chopped onion
- 1 1/4 cups shredded Cheddar cheese, divided

Instructions:

1. Lightly grease the slow cooker with cooking oil.
2. Mix together the egg, cottage cheese, butter, onion, flour, 1 cup of cheddar cheese, and broccoli in the slow cooker.
3. Cover the slow cooker and cook for 1 hour on high, then stir up the ingredients and put the heat to low.
4. Cover and cook for 2 hours and 30 minutes, then top with the rest of the cheddar cheese. Serve warm.

Arianna Brooks

Mexican Breakfast Casserole

Makes: 5 servings

Carbs per serving: 5.2 grams

Ingredients:

- 6 ounce pork sausage roll
- ½ teaspoon garlic powder
- ½ teaspoon coriander powder
- ½ teaspoon cumin powder
- ½ teaspoon chili powder
- Salt to taste
- Pepper powder to taste
- ½ cup low fat milk
- ½ cup cheese of your choice
- Sour cream (optional)
- Avocado (optional)
- Salsa (optional)
- 1 tablespoon cilantro (optional)

Instructions:

1. Place a skillet over medium heat. Add the sausage. Cook for a few minutes until it is no longer pink.
2. Add salsa salt, pepper, chili powder, and cumin and coriander powders. Mix well and remove from heat.
3. Whisk together eggs and milk in a large bowl. Add the pork and cheese. Mix well.
4. Transfer into a greased slow cooker.
5. Cover the pot and cook on low for 5 hours or on high for 2 ½ hours.
6. Serve with toppings if desired.

Italian Beef Sandwiches

Makes: 4 servings

Carbs per serving: 8 grams

Ingredients:

- 1 ¼ pound grass fed beef chuck roast
- ½ tablespoon olive oil
- ½ teaspoon dried basil
- ½ teaspoon dried oregano
- ½ teaspoon dried crushed rosemary
- 1 teaspoon garlic powder
- 2 teaspoons onion powder
- Salt to taste
- Black pepper powder to taste
- ¼ cup water
- ½ tablespoon red wine vinegar
- 1 tablespoon Dijon mustard
- 4 large Portobello mushroom caps

Instructions:

1. Mix together all the dry ingredients and rub it on to the chuck roast.
2. Place a skillet over medium heat. Add oil. When the oil is heated, add the roast. Cook 4-5 minutes per side.
3. Transfer the roast into the slow cooker. Add water and vinegar.
4. Cover the pot and cook on low for 7-8 hours.
5. When done, remove the beef and shred the beef with fork.

6. Remove any fat that is left behind in the pot. Add Dijon mustard to the remaining juices in the pot and mix well.
7. Add the shredded beef back to the pot and mix well.
8. To make the buns: Place the Portobello mushrooms on a baking sheet. Sprinkle salt, pepper and a little olive oil. Bake in a preheated oven at 450 degree F for about 10 minutes.
9. Place the beef over the mushroom buns and serve.

Slow Cooked Breakfast Pizza

Makes: 16servings

Carbs per serving: 7.6 grams

Ingredients:

- 1 ½ pound ground beef, cooked,
- 1 ½ pound bulk Italian sausage, cooked
- 2 jars (15 ounce each) pizza sauce
- 6 cups mozzarella cheese, shredded
- 6 cups fresh spinach
- 32 slices pepperoni
- 2 cups olives, sliced
- 2 cups mushrooms, sliced
- 1 green pepper, chopped
- 1 cup onions, chopped
- 4 cloves garlic, minced

Instructions:

1. Mix together sausage, ground beef, pizza sauce, and onions.
2. Add half of this mixture to the pot of the slow cooker. Lay half of the spinach leaves over the mixture. Lay half of the pepperoni over the spinach. Sprinkle half of each of the following - olives, peppers, garlic, mushrooms, and mozzarella cheese.
3. Repeat step 2 with the remaining ingredients.
4. Close the pot and cook on low for 6-8 hours.
5. When done, cool it slightly and slice into 16 pieces.
6. Left over slices can be refrigerated and reheated.

Arianna Brooks

Breakfast Casserole

Makes: 4 servings

Carbs per serving: 8 grams with hashed brown

Carbs per serving: 4.8 grams without hashed brown

Ingredients:

- 2 cups hashed brown Jicama OR Daikon radish hashed brown (optional)
- 6 ounce package cooked bacon slices, crumbled
- ½ pound cooked, drained ground sausage
- 1 small yellow onions, diced
- ½ a green bell pepper, diced
- ¾ cup fresh mushrooms, sliced
- 1 cup fresh spinach
- 1 cup shredded Monterrey Jack cheese
- 1/4 cup feta cheese, chopped
- 6 eggs
- ½ cup heavy white cream
- ½ teaspoon salt or to taste
- ½ teaspoon pepper powder or to taste

Instructions:

1. Spread the hash browns on the bottom of the slow cooker.
2. Lay the bacon over it followed by layers of sausages, onions, bell pepper, spinach, mushroom, and cheese.
3. Beat together in a bowl, eggs, cream, salt, and pepper. Pour this mixture all over in the crock-pot.
4. Cover the cooker and cook on low for 8-10 hours.

Burrito

Makes: 8 servings

Carbs per serving: 6 grams

Ingredients:

- 3 pounds lean pork, boneless, cubed
- 24 ounce diced tomatoes with green chilies
- 1 large onion, diced
- 2 jalapeno, diced
- 1 teaspoon ground chipotle
- ½ teaspoon cayenne pepper
- ½ teaspoon ground jalapeno
- 4 cloves garlic minced
- Few large lettuce leaves

Instructions:

1. Add all the ingredients except the lettuce to the pot of the slow cooker. Mix well.
2. Cook on low for about 7-8 hours. When done mix well.
3. Divide this filling among the lettuce leaves, roll and serve.

Arianna Brooks

Mushroom and Basil Egg Pie

Makes: 8 servings

Carbs per serving: 11 grams

Ingredients:

- 1 cup egg or egg substitute
- 1/8 cup all-purpose flour
- 1/8 tsp salt
- 1/8 tsp pepper
- 1/6 tsp baking powder
- 4 oz. low fat Monterrey Jack cheese, shredded
- 1/2 cup sliced mushrooms
- 1/2 cup low fat large curd cottage cheese
- 1/3 tsp dried basil leaves

Instructions:

1. Mix together the flour, salt, pepper, and baking powder.
2. In a bowl, whisk the eggs until foamy, then gradually whisk in the flour mixture until thoroughly incorporated. Add the remaining ingredients and mix well.
3. Lightly grease the slow cooker with cooking oil, then pour the egg and mushroom mixture into it. Cover and cook for 4 hours on low.
4. Turn off the heat and let it stand for about 5 minutes before inverting the pie onto a plate. Slice, then serve.

Cauliflower Hash Browns Casserole

Makes: 4 servings

Carbs per serving: 5.7 grams

Ingredients:
- 6 eggs
- ¼ cup milk
- ½ teaspoon dry mustard
- Salt to taste
- Pepper powder to taste
- 1 medium head cauliflower, shredded
- 1 small onion, chopped
- 5 ounce package cooked sausages, sliced
- 1 cup cheddar cheese, shredded
- Cooking spray

Instructions:
1. Spray the slow cooker pot with cooking spray.
2. In a bowl, add eggs, milk, mustard, salt and pepper. Whisk well.
3. Place half the cauliflower at the bottom of the pot. Spread well. Next sprinkle half the onions. Sprinkle salt and pepper. Lay half the sausages and half the cheese over the sausages.
4. Repeat step 3 with the remaining half ingredients.
5. Pour the beaten egg mixture all over the cooker pot.
6. Cover and cook on low for 5-7 hours or until the top is golden brown.

Arianna Brooks

Egg & Sausage Breakfast Casserole

Makes: 6 to 8 servings

Carbs per serving: 5.89 grams

Ingredients:

- 10 eggs
- 1 medium-sized broccoli heads, chopped
- 1 12-oz pack sausages, cooked and sliced
- 1 cup cheddar cheese, shredded, divided
- 3/4 cup whipping cream
- 2 cloves garlic, minced
- 1/4 tsp pepper
- 1/2 tsp salt

Instructions:

1. Get a 6-quart slow cooker and grease its ceramic interior well.
2. Lay half the broccoli, half the cheese, and half the sausages in the slow cooker. Do the same with the rest of the broccoli, cheese, and sausages.
3. Whisk together the eggs, garlic, whipping cream, salt & pepper until everything is well combined. Pour on top of the layered ingredients.
4. Cover the pot and cook under low heat setting for about 4 to 5 hours or 2 to 3 hours under high heat setting, until the edges are browned and all set at the center.
5. Transfer to a serving dish. Serve and enjoy!

Frittata w/ Roasted Red Pepper, Artichoke Hearts, & Feta

Makes: 6 servings

Carbs per serving: 9 grams

Ingredients:

- 14 oz. (1 can) artichoke hearts, small, drained and cut into tiny pieces (or pre-cut artichokes)
- 12 oz. (1 jar) roasted red peppers, drained & cut into tiny pieces
- 1/4 cup green onions, sliced
- 8 eggs, well-beaten or until whites and yolks are combined completely
- 4 oz. feta cheese, crumbled
- 1 tsp seasoning to taste
- Black pepper, fresh-ground to taste
- 2 tsp parsley, chopped for garnish (optional)

Instructions:

1. Place the artichoke hearts in a colander and let them drain them well in the sink. Meanwhile, you can crumble the feta and slice the onions. Spray the insert of the slow cooker with non-stick spray very well.
2. Remove the artichoke hearts from the colander and in their place, allow the roasted red peppers to drain. Chop the artichoke hearts into quarters, or even smaller if they are large. Place the artichoke pieces at the bottom of cooker insert. Next, cut the red peppers (drained) into approximately ½" squares and add them into the cooker. Put the green onions next.

3. Beat the eggs well or until the yolks and whites are thoroughly blended, then pour the beaten eggs over the veggies in the slow cooker. Gently stir with a fork to distribute the pieces of artichoke, green onions, and red pepper well. Drizzle with crumbled feta on top, then put some seasoning. Add the freshly ground black pepper.
4. Allow to cook for 2 to 3 hours or until the eggs reach the desired firmness, and when the cheese is completely melted.
5. Cut the frittata into smaller pieces while still inside the slow cooker. Remove the cut pieces.
6. Sprinkle and garnish with parsley, if desired.
7. Serve hot and enjoy.

Slow Cooker Low Carb

Egg, Bacon and Hash Brown Casserole

Makes: 8 servings

Carbs per serving: 14 gram

Ingredients:

- 20 oz. bag shredded hash browns, frozen
- 8 slices bacon, thick-cut, cooked and chopped coarsely
- 8 oz. cheddar cheese, shredded
- 6 green onions, sliced thinly
- 12 eggs
- 1/2 cup milk
- 1/2 tsp salt
- 1/4 tsp pepper
- Cooking oil (to coat slow cooker lightly)

Instructions:

1. Grease the slow cooker lightly with cooking oil. Layer the bottom of the cooker with half of the hash browns topped with half of the bacon, 1/3 of the green onions, and ½ of the cheese. Set some bacon and green onions aside for garnishing. Repeat the process with a 2nd layer of hash browns, bacon, onion, and cheese.
2. Get a large-sized bowl, and whisk the milk, eggs, and salt & pepper together. Slowly pour the mix over the top. Allow to cook until the eggs are set, or about 2 to 3 hours over high heat setting or 4 to 5 hours over low heat. Sprinkle the rest of the onions and bacon on top.
3. Serve with or without hot sauce (depending on preference) immediately.

Arianna Brooks

Breakfast Meatloaf

Makes: 4 servings

Carbs per serving: 8 grams

Ingredients:

- 2 lbs. ground pork
- 2 eggs
- 3 cloves garlic, minced
- 1 onion, diced
- 1 tbsp. coconut oil
- 1 tsp red pepper, crushed & flaked
- 2 tsp of sea salt
- 1 tbsp. sage, fresh, minced
- 1 tsp dried oregano
- 1 tbsp. smoked paprika
- 1/4 cup of almond flour
- 1 tsp of marjoram

Instructions:

Heat coconut oil on medium-high setting. Add and sauté the onions until soft.

1. Put in the garlic and sauté for 3 to 4 minutes or until fragrance comes out.
2. Remove the spices from the heat and set aside to allow them to cool slightly.
3. Combine the pork and the rest of the ingredients in a mixing bowl.
4. Include the garlic and onion.

5. Using your clean hands, evenly blend everything. Make sure not to over mix; otherwise, the meatloaf might get tough and mealy as it cooks.
6. Move the pork over to the slow cooker. Then make a loaf shape. See to it that the meatloaf does not touch any of the sides.
7. Turn the slow cooker on and allow to cook for about 3 hours on low heat setting; make sure not to let it stay on warm, as it will cause the meatloaf to dry out.
8. Let the meatloaf cool a little before slicing.
9. Transfer the dish into an airtight container.
10. The following morning put a small amount of oil in a skillet and heat on medium high setting.
11. Put a slice of meatloaf in the skillet and let it brown on each side.
12. Remove from the skillet and transfer to a serving dish.
13. Enjoy while hot.

Arianna Brooks

Slow Cooker Bacon, Egg & Hash Brown Casserole

Makes: 8 servings

Carbs per serving: 14 grams

Ingredients:

- 8 slices thick-cut cooked and coarsely chopped bacon
- 12 eggs
- 20 ounce bag shredded hash browns (frozen)
- 6 thinly sliced green onions
- 1/2 cup milk
- 8 ounces cheddar cheese (shredded)
- 1/2 teaspoon salt
- Cooking oil (for coating)
- 1/4 teaspoon pepper

Instructions:

1. Grease the slow cooker with cooking oil- light greasing should do.
2. Spread half of the hash browns in the bottom of the cooker.
3. Top the hash browns layer with half the bacon, followed by half the cheese.
4. Finally spread one-third of the sliced green onions.
5. Repeat this with the second layer in the same format (hash browns first, bacon next, followed by cheese and green onions).
6. Reserve some green onions and bacon for garnishing.
7. Take a large and crack the eggs into it.
8. Add milk, pepper and salt to the cracked eggs.

9. Beat the mixture thoroughly or you can whisk it until well-combined
10. Pour this egg-milk mixture over the hash-bacon-cheese-onion mix in the cooker
11. Let it cook for 3 hours on high or 5 hours on low until the eggs are completely set
12. Spring the reserved onions and bacon over the top.
13. Serve warm and enjoy!

Arianna Brooks

Slow Cooker Frittata with Artichoke Hearts, Roasted Red Pepper, and Feta

Makes: 8 servings

Carbs per serving: 9 grams

Ingredients:

- 8 beaten eggs (yolks and whites should be well-combined)
- 12 ounces roasted red peppers (drained and sliced into small pieces)
- 14 ounces small cut artichoke hearts (drained)
- 1 teaspoon fresh-ground black pepper
- 1/4 cup green onions (sliced)
- 1 teaspoon all-purpose seasoning will work
- 4 ounces Feta cheese (crumbled)
- 2 tablespoons parsley (chopped)
- Nonstick cooking spray

Instructions:

1. Drain the artichoke hearts using a colander, finely slice the green onions and crumble the feta cheese. Set aside.
2. Grease the slow cooker insert with a nonstick cooking spray
3. If you haven't brought the already-cut artichoke hearts, then you can chop them into small quarters.
4. Drain the roasted red peppers using a colander and slice them into small pieces
5. Layer the chopped artichoke hearts in the bottom of the slow cooker.

6. Top it with the chopped red peppers and then layer the green onions over it.
7. If you haven't already beaten the eggs ready, crack the eggs in a large bowl. Use an immersion blender to beat the eggs well until the yolks and whites are thoroughly combined.
8. Pour this egg mixture over the layered artichoke-red pepper-onion mixture in the slow cooker
9. Gently stir the mixture with a fork or spoon to make sure the artichoke, red pepper and green onion pieces are properly distributed
10. Now, sprinkle the crumbled feta cheese over the top and season it with all-purpose seasoning powder and ground pepper.
11. Allow it to cook for 3 hours on low until the cheese is melted and the eggs are firmly set.
12. Cut the frittata into pieces while it is still in the slow cooker
13. Garnish with chopped parsley and serve warm.

Arianna Brooks

Slow Cooker Kale Bacon Breakfast Casserole

Makes: 4 servings

Carbs per serving: 4 grams

Ingredients:

- 3 large bacon slices (around 3.2 ounces)
- 6 eggs (large ones)
- 1 cup chopped white mushrooms (around 2.5 ounces)
- 3 tablespoons shallots (chopped)
- 8 large kale leaves (shredded finely)
- 1/2 cup chopped red bell pepper (around 2.7 ounces)
- 1 cup Parmesan cheese (shredded)
- 1 tablespoon butter
- 1 tablespoon finely chopped spinach
- 1 sliced avocado dressed in extra-virgin olive oil
- Salt and pepper, to taste
- 2 tablespoons olive oil

Instructions:

1. Wash the kale, remove the hard stems and chop into fine pieces. You can also shred the leaves using the food processor
2. Heat the olive oil over medium heat in the large saucepan and add the bacon slices to it
3. Cook until the bacon is crispy.
4. Add the mushrooms, shallots and the red pepper to the cooker. Sauté until the contents soften.
5. Add the shredded kale leaves and mix well. Turn off the heat after 10 seconds and let it sit until the kale wilts

6. Take a large bowl and crack the eggs. Add salt and pepper to the cracked eggs.
7. Beat it well until they are combined well
8. Turn on the slow cooker and set it high. Place the butter in the cooker and allow it to melt.
9. Brush the inside of the cooker with the melted butter until completely greased.
10. Transfer the sautéed vegetable-bacon mixture to the base of the slow cooker.
11. Sprinkle the cheese over the veggie meat mixture and pour the beaten eggs on top
12. Stir the contents well until the flavors blend and the ingredients are well incorporated
13. Cook on high for 1.5 hours or on low for 6 hours.
14. Transfer the casserole to a place and garnish with chopped spinach and avocado dressed with oil. Serve warm and enjoy!

Arianna Brooks

Breakfast Casserole with Cheese and Sausage (Gluten free)

Makes: 9 servings

Carbs per serving: 0.9 grams

Ingredients:

- 2 cups Cheddar cheese, divided
- 1 pound breakfast sausage
- 12 eggs (large ones)
- 3 cups broccoli (washed, drained and cut into florets)
- 6 minced garlic cloves
- 2 tablespoons chopped fresh parsley + extra for garnish
- 1/2 cup heavy cream
- 1/4 teaspoon black pepper
- 1/4 teaspoon sea salt
- 1 teaspoon olive oil
- Nonstick cooking spray

Instructions:

1. Heat the oil in a skillet over medium heat and add the minced garlic to it.
2. Cook for a minute until the raw flavor goes and you get the fragrance
3. Add the breakfast sausage to the skillet and sauté for 5 minutes until lightly browned. As you brown, use a spatula to break the sausages
4. Take a large bowl and crack the eggs. Add half the Cheddar cheese, heavy cream, black pepper, parsley and sea salt to it.
5. Whisk together until they are well-combined

6. Grease the inside of the slow cooker with a nonstick cooking spray.
7. Spread the crumbled sautéed sausage in the bottom of the slow cooker
8. Top it with broccoli in the next layer as you evenly spread the florets
9. Pour the egg-cream mixture over the top and sprinkle with the remaining cheddar cheese.
10. Cook on high for 1.5 to 2 hours until the cheese melts and the eggs are firmly set
11. Transfer the casserole to a plate and sprinkle with chopped parsley
12. Serve warm and enjoy!

Arianna Brooks

Slow Cooker Frittata with Kale, Roasted Red Pepper, and Feta

Makes: 8 servings

Carbs per serving: 6 grams

Ingredients:

- 5 ounces baby kale
- 6 ounces roasted red pepper (diced small)
- 5 ounces crumbled Feta cheese
- 8 well beaten eggs
- 1/4 cup green onion (sliced)
- 2 teaspoons olive oil (to sauté the kale)
- Low-fat sour cream (for serving)
- Non-stick cooking spray
- 1 teaspoon black pepper (freshly ground)
- 1/2 teaspoon all-purpose seasoning blend

Instructions:

1. Wash the kale well, remove the stems, drain and pat them dry with a paper towel.
2. Heat the 2 tablespoons olive oil in a large skillet over medium heat and add the kale leaves to the skillet
3. Sauté until the kale leaves wilts and softens
4. Grease the slow cooker insert with a nonstick cooking spray
5. Layer the sautéed kale leaves in the bottom of the slow cooker
6. Drain the roasted red peppers using a colander and slice them into small pieces

7. Top the kale leaves with the chopped red peppers and then, layer the green onions over it.
8. If you haven't already beaten the eggs ready, crack the eggs in a large bowl. Use an immersion blender to beat the eggs well until the yolks and whites are thoroughly combined.
9. Pour this egg mixture over the layered kale-red pepper-onion mixture in the slow cooker
10. Gently stir the mixture with a fork or spoon to make sure the kale, red pepper and green onion pieces are properly distributed
11. Now, sprinkle the crumbled feta cheese over the top and season it with all-purpose seasoning powder and ground pepper.
12. Allow it to cook for 2 hours on low until the cheese is melted and the eggs are firmly set.
13. Cut the frittata into pieces while it is still in the slow cooker.
14. Transfer to a plate and serve with a dollop of sour cream. Enjoy!

Arianna Brooks

Greek Eggs Breakfast Casserole

Makes: 6 servings

Carbs per serving: 7 grams

Ingredients:

- 12 whisked eggs
- 1/2 cup sun dried tomatoes packed in oil (chopped)
- 1 cup sliced baby Bella mushrooms
- 1 tablespoon finely chopped red onion
- 2 cups spinach (chopped)
- 1/2 cup Feta Cheese (crumbled)
- 1/2 cup milk
- 1 teaspoon minced garlic
- 1 teaspoon black pepper
- 1/2 teaspoon salt
- Nonstick cooking spray
- 1 tablespoon chopped parsley

Instructions:

1. Take a large bowl and place the already whisked eggs in it
2. Add milk, pepper and salt to the whisked eggs.
3. Whisk them together until well-combined and add the minced garlic along with chopped onions
4. Now, add the chopped sundried tomatoes, sliced mushrooms and chopped spinach to the bowl.
5. Mix them well until well combined.
6. Grease the inside of a slow cooker with a nonstick cooking spray

7. Pour the egg-milk mixture to the bottom of the cooker and sprinkle the crumbled cheese over the top
8. Let it cook on low for 3-4 hours until the cheese melts and the eggs are cooked
9. Transfer to a plate and garnish with chopped parsley
10. Serve warm and enjoy!

Arianna Brooks

Slow Cooker Veggie Omelet

Makes: 4 servings

Carbs per serving: 8 grams

Ingredients:

- 1 finely chopped yellow onion (small one should do)
- 6 eggs (large ones)
- 1/2 cup milk
- 1 thinly sliced red bell pepper
- 1 minced garlic clove
- 1 cup broccoli florets
- 1/8 teaspoon chili powder
- 1/4 teaspoon salt
- 1/8 teaspoon garlic powder
- 1 teaspoon pepper (freshly ground)
- Nonstick cooking spray

For Garnishing

- 1 tablespoon shredded cheddar cheese
- 1 tablespoon chopped tomatoes
- 1 tablespoon chopped onions
- 1 tablespoon fresh parsley

Instructions:

1. Grease the inside of the slow cooking with a nonstick cooking spray and set it aside
2. Take a large bowl and crack the eggs.
3. Add milk, garlic powder, pepper, chili powder and salt to the cracked eggs

Slow Cooker Low Carb

4. Whisk together the mixture until well-combined (use an egg beater or immersion blender)
5. Now add the sliced red peppers, minced garlic, chopped onions and broccoli florets to the greased slow cooker
6. Pour the egg-milk mixture over it and stir the contents until well-combined
7. Let it cook on high for 2 hours. Check once after 1.5 hours to see if the eggs are set and the omelet is done.
8. Once the 2 hours cooking cycle is over sprinkle the shredded cheese over the omelet.
9. Cover the cooker and let it sit for 5 minutes until the cheese melts over the egg
10. Turn off the cooker and slice the omelet into eight wedges.
11. Transfer to a plate and garnish with chopped onions, chopped tomatoes and chopped parsley.
12. Serve warm and enjoy!

Arianna Brooks

Chapter Four - Main Course – Beef

Layered Brisket Dinner with Tangy Mustard Sauce

Makes: 4 servings

Carbs per serving: 14 grams

Ingredients:

For tangy mustard sauce

- ¼ cup light sour cream
- ¼ teaspoon Italian seasoning
- ¼ teaspoon fresh thyme (optional)
- ¾ teaspoon Dijon style mustard

For brisket

- 1 ½ pounds beef brisket, trimmed of fat
- ½ tablespoon Worcestershire sauce
- Black pepper powder to taste
- 4 ounces baby carrots
- 1 teaspoon olive oil
- Salt to taste
- Snipped fresh thyme (optional)
- ½ tablespoon Dijon style mustard
- ½ tablespoon balsamic vinegar
- ½ pound baby red or yellow potatoes, halved if large
- ½ small onion, cut into wedges
- ¼ teaspoon dried Italian seasoning, crushed

Instructions:

1. To make tangy mustard sauce: Add sour cream, thyme, Italian seasoning and mustard into a bowl and whisk until well combined.
2. Cover and refrigerate until use.
3. To make layered brisket: Lay the brisket in the slow cooker.
4. Add mustard, vinegar, pepper powder and Worcestershire sauce into a bowl and whisk well. Spoon the sauce mixture over the brisket. Turn the brisket and spoon the sauce mixture on the other side too. Spread the mixture.
5. Take a large sheet of heavy foil. Lay carrots, potato and onion over it. Trickle oil over the vegetables and season with salt, pepper and Italian seasoning. Take one side of the foil and fold it over the vegetables so as to cover them. Repeat with the remaining sides. Seal completely and place in the slow cooker, over the brisket.
6. Cover the pot and cook on Low for 8-9 hours.
7. Remove brisket from the pot and place on your cutting board. When cool enough to handle, cut into slices.
8. Unfold the foil packet just before serving.
9. Divide brisket slices into 4 plates. Divide the vegetables and place on the plates. Serve with tangy mustard sauce.

Slow Cooker Low Carb

Boeuf Bourguignon with Spiralized Vegetables

Makes: 3 servings

Carbs per serving: 6 grams

Ingredients:

- 1 ½ pounds beef chuck roast, round roast, cut into 1 inch cubes
- 2 ½ slices bacon, cubed
- Salt to taste
- Black pepper powder to taste
- 2 stalks celery, chopped
- ½ tablespoon tomato paste
- 2 sprigs fresh thyme
- ½ cup chicken broth or beef broth, or more if required
- 1 medium carrot, peeled
- 1 medium onion
- 2 cloves garlic, minced
- ½ pound white button mushrooms, sliced
- 1 bay leaf
- Red pepper flakes to taste
- ½ cup red wine
- A handful fresh parsley, chopped, to garnish

Instructions:

1. Make noodles of the onion and carrots using blade A of the spiralizer. Set aside.
2. Place a skillet over medium high heat. Add bacon and cook until crisp. Remove bacon with a slotted spoon and place over a plate lined with paper towels.

3. Sprinkle salt and pepper generously over the beef. Add beef into the skillet. Spread in a single layer. Cook in batches if necessary.
4. Cook for 2-3 minutes or until light brown. Flip sides and cook the other side until light brown. Transfer into the slow cooker.
5. Add spiralized onion noodles, bacon, celery, mushroom, bay leaf, thyme sprigs and garlic into the pot and stir.
6. Cover the pot and cook on High for 3 hours. Add carrot noodles when the meat is tender. Cook for some more time until the meat is coming off the bones.
7. When done, discard bay leaves and thyme.
8. Ladle into bowls. Garnish with parsley and serve.

Slow Cooker Picadillo

Makes: 5-6 servings (½ cup each)

Carbs per serving: 5 grams (without brown rice or cauliflower rice)

Ingredients:

- 1 ¼ pounds 93% lean ground beef
- ½ cup red bell pepper, chopped
- ½ cup onions, minced
- 2 tablespoons cilantro, chopped
- 2 cloves garlic, minced
- 4 oz. canned tomato sauce
- ½ small tomato, chopped
- 2 tablespoons alcaparrado (mixture of manzanilla olives, pimientos, capers) or green olives
- 1 bay leaf
- 1 teaspoon ground cumin
- Freshly ground black pepper to taste
- 1/8 teaspoon garlic powder
- Kosher salt to taste
- ¾ -1 cup water

Instructions:

1. Place a skillet over medium heat. Sprinkle salt and pepper generously over the beef and place in the skillet. Cook until brown. Break it simultaneously as it cooks.
2. Cook until the beef is not pink anymore. Drain the fat from the pan.
3. Stir in the onion, garlic and bell pepper and stir-fry for a couple of minutes. Turn off the heat and add all the ingredients from the skillet into the slow cooker.

4. Stir in rest of the ingredients.
5. Cover the pot and cook on low for 5-7 hours or on high for 2 ½ -3 ½ hours. Taste and adjust the salt if necessary. Discard the bay leaf.
6. Serve over brown rice or cauliflower rice.

Beef Curry

Makes: 8 servings

Carbs per serving: 15 grams (without brown rice or cauliflower rice)

Ingredients:

- 2 pounds lean stew meat
- 2 small sweet onions, chopped
- 4 teaspoons fresh ginger, grated
- Black pepper powder to taste
- 4 cloves garlic, chopped
- 3 ½ cups beef broth or stock
- Sea salt to taste
- 4 teaspoons curry powder
- 1 cup fresh cilantro, chopped (optional)
- 2 tablespoons arrowroot powder mixed with 2 tablespoons water

Instructions:

1. Season beef with curry powder and place in the slow cooker. Scatter rest of the ingredients except cilantro and arrowroot mixture over the meat and mix until well incorporated.
2. Cover the pot and cook on Low for 5-6 hours or until meat is cooked. Add cornstarch mixture during the last 12-15 minutes of cooking.
3. Stir and serve over cauliflower rice or brown rice.

Arianna Brooks

Pepperoni Pizza Chili

Makes: 3 servings

Carbs per serving: 10 grams

Ingredients:

- ¼ hot Italian style turkey sausage
- ¾ pound 95% lean ground beef
- 2 oz. sliced turkey pepperoni, sliced in half
- ½ cup onion, chopped
- 4 oz. marinara sauce
- ¼ cup water
- 2 cloves garlic, minced
- 1 small green bell pepper, chopped
- 4 oz. Salsa
- ½ teaspoon dried oregano
- ½ teaspoon chili powder or to taste
- Black pepper powder to taste
- Salt to taste
- 1/3 cup part skim mozzarella cheese

Instructions:

1. Place a Dutch oven over medium heat. Add beef, sausage, garlic, onion and bell pepper. Cook until the meat is not pink anymore. Break the meat simultaneously as it cooks. Drain the excess fat if required and transfer meat into the slow cooker.
2. Add marinara sauce, salsa, pepperoni, water, salt, oregano, pepper and chili powder and mix well.
3. Cover the pot and cook on Low for 4-6 hours or on High for 2-4 hours.

4. Ladle into bowls and serve.

Crockpot Bolognese

Makes: 10 servings (½ cup each)

Carbs per serving: 5 grams (without noodles)

Ingredients:

- 2 oz. pancetta, chopped or center cut bacon
- 1 medium white onion, minced
- 1 pound 95% lean ground beef
- 1 medium carrot, minced
- 2 tablespoons white wine
- 2 bay leaves
- 2 tablespoons fresh parsley, chopped
- ½ tablespoon butter or olive oil
- 1 celery stalk, minced
- 1 can (28 ounces) crushed tomatoes
- Salt to taste
- Pepper to taste
- ¼ cup half and half

Instructions:

1. Place a skillet over low heat. Add pancetta and cook until fat is released.
2. Stir in the butter, celery, onions and carrots and cook until slightly tender.
3. Raise the heat to medium high. Add beef, salt and pepper and cook until brown. Drain excess fat in the pan.
4. Stir in the wine. Cook until it is reduced to half its original quantity. Turn off the heat.

5. Add tomatoes, salt, pepper and bay leaves into the slow cooker. Transfer meat into a slow cooker. Mix well.
6. Cover the pot and cook on Low for 5-6 hours.
7. Taste and adjust the seasoning if necessary. Stir in half and half of parsley.
8. Serve over low carb noodles of your choice.

Slow Cooked Beef with Carrots and Cabbage

Makes: 4 servings

Carbs per serving: 14 grams

Ingredients:

- 16 oz. beef chuck roast, boneless
- ½ teaspoon ground cumin
- Salt to taste
- ½ teaspoon dried oregano, crushed
- Black pepper powder to taste
- ½ teaspoon paprika
- Nonstick cooking spray
- 4 small cloves garlic, minced
- 4 cups green cabbage, shredded
- 6 medium carrots, cut into 2 inch pieces
- 2/3 cup beef broth

Instructions:

1. Add cumin, oregano, pepper, salt and paprika into a bowl and whisk well. Mix well and rub this mixture over the roast.
2. Place a nonstick skillet over medium heat. Spray some cooking spray over it.
3. Add roast and cook until brown.
4. Add carrots, garlic and broth into the slow cooker. Place roast over the carrots.
5. Cover the pot and cook on Low for 6 to 7 hours or on high for 3 to 4 hours.
6. Add cabbage and cook for 30 minutes.

7. Remove meat with a slotted spoon and place on your cutting board. When cool enough to handle, cut into slices.
8. Serve meat with carrot and cabbage.

Slow Cooker Chipotle Beef Barbacoa

Makes: 9 servings

Carbs per serving: 2 grams

Ingredients:

- 3 pounds chuck roast or Beef brisket (trimmed and cut into 2-inch chunks)
- 2 medium Chipotle chilies in adobo (including 4 teaspoons of sauce)
- 1/2 cup chicken broth or beef broth
- 1/2 teaspoon cloves (ground)
- 5 minced garlic cloves
- 1 tablespoon dried oregano
- 2 tablespoons apple cider vinegar
- 2 whole Bay leaf
- 2 tablespoons lime juice
- 1 teaspoon black pepper
- 2 teaspoons cumin
- 2 teaspoons sea salt
- Nonstick cooking spray

Instructions:

1. Take a high-speed blender and add the chipotle chilies in adobe sauce, chicken broth, ground cloves, minced garlic, dried oregano, apple cider vinegar, lime juice, black pepper, cumin and sea salt to it.
2. Blend on high for 60 seconds until the contents get into a smooth, creamy puree consistency

3. Lightly grease the insides of the slow cooker with a nonstick cooking spray and place the beef pieces in the bottom of the cooker.
4. Pour the blended puree from the blender over the beef chucks.
5. Place the entire bay leaves over the top.
6. Cook on high for 6 hours or cook on low for 10 hours until the beef becomes tender such that they fall apart easily.
7. Remove the bay leaves and use two forks to shred the nicely cooked meat.
8. Stir the shredded meat well with the liquid juice in the slow cooker.
9. Cover the cooker and let it rest for 10 minutes for the meat to absorb more flavor.
10. Transfer to a plate and serve warm

Slow Cooker Low Carb

Hungarian Beef Goulash

Makes: 8 servings

Carbs per serving: 6 grams

Ingredients:

- 2 pounds trimmed and cubed beef stew meat (chuck or similar)
- 14 ounces reduced-sodium beef broth (1 can)
- 1 teaspoon Worcestershire sauce
- 1 chopped large onion (or 2 medium onions)
- 14 ounces diced tomatoes (1 can)
- 3 minced garlic cloves
- 1 chopped small red bell pepper
- 2 tablespoons sweet or hot Hungarian paprika (or you can mix 1 tablespoon sweet paprika with 1 tablespoon hot paprika)
- 1 tablespoon cornstarch + 2 tablespoons water (mix and keep ready)
- 2 teaspoons caraway seeds (crushed)
- 2 tablespoons fresh parsley (chopped)
- 1/4 teaspoon salt
- 2 bay leaves
- Freshly ground pepper, to taste
- Nonstick cooking spray

Instructions:

1. Lightly grease the inside of the slow cooker with nonstick cooking spray
2. Place the beef stew meat in the bottom of slow cooker and set aside

3. Take a small bowl and combine the crushed caraway seeds, salt, pepper and paprika until mixed well
4. Sprinkle this spice mixture over the beef in the cooker and toss it well until coated completely.
5. Add the bell pepper and onion to the slow cooker. Give the contents a quick stir and set aside
6. Take a medium skillet and combine the broth, Worcestershire sauce, tomatoes and garlic in it.
7. Cook the contents over medium heat and bring it to simmer.
8. Turn off heat and pour this mixture over the beef-bell pepper-onion mixture in the slow cooker
9. Place the bay leaves over the top and cover the cooker
10. Cook on high for 4.5 hours or on low for 7.5 hours until the meat becomes soft and tender
11. Once the cooking cycle is done, remove the bay leaves
12. If you see any visible fat over the stew surface, blot or skim it and add the prepared cornstarch mixture to it.
13. Cook on high for 15 minutes stirring frequently until the liquid thickens.
14. Transfer to a plate and sprinkle the parsley.
15. Serve warm and enjoy!

Slow-Cooker Braised Beef with Carrots & Turnips

Makes: 8 servings

Carbs per serving: 13 grams

Ingredients:

- 3 pounds trimmed beef chuck roast
- 2 peeled medium turnips (cut into half-inch pieces)
- 5 peeled medium carrots (cut into half-inch pieces)
- 1 chopped medium onion
- 28 ounces whole tomatoes (1 can)
- 3 sliced garlic cloves
- 1 cup red wine
- 2 tablespoons extra-virgin olive oil
- 1/2 teaspoon ground pepper
- 1 tablespoon kosher salt
- 2 teaspoons ground cinnamon
- 1/4 teaspoon ground cloves
- 1/2 teaspoon ground allspice
- Chopped fresh basil, for garnishing
- Nonstick cooking spray

Instructions:

1. Take a small bowl and combine the allspice, cloves, cinnamon, pepper and salt together until mixed well.
2. Rub this spice mixture all over the meat and set aside.
3. Heat oil over medium heat in a large skillet and add beef to it.
4. Cook for 5 minutes on each side until the meat is browned.

5. Grease the inside of the slow cooker with a nonstick cooking spray and transfer the browned meat from the skillet to the cooker.
6. Add the garlic and onion to the same skillet. Continue to cook for another 2 minutes stirring in between.
7. Add the tomatoes with their juice and pour the wine over to the garlic-onion-tomato mixture in the skillet.
8. Bring the contents to boil while you scrape up the browned bits in the bottom of the skillet.
9. Break the tomatoes while you stir and let it cook until the mixture thickens
10. Add this mixture over the meat into the slow cooker.
11. Add the turnips and carrots to the contents in the cooker.
12. Cover the cooker and cook on high for 4 hours or on low for 8 hours
13. After the cooking cycle, remove the cooked beef from the cooker and transfer it to plate.
14. Slice the meat with a sharp knife or fork. Pour the sauce (cooking liquid from slow cooker) over the meat.
15. Serve with the vegetables (in the cooker) and garnish with basil.
16. Relish and enjoy!

Fireside Beef Stew

Makes: 6 servings

Carbs per serving: 15 grams

Ingredients:

- 1 1/2 pounds beef chuck pot roast (boneless)
- 9 ounces frozen Italian green beans (1 package)
- 2 small onions (cut into wedges)
- 2 tablespoons Worcestershire sauce
- 4 teaspoons cornstarch
- 2 tablespoons cold water
- 1 pound peeled and seeded butternut squash (cut into 1-inch pieces)
- 14 ounces reduced-sodium beef broth (1 can)
- 2 minced garlic cloves
- 1 teaspoon dry mustard
- 8 ounces tomato sauce (1 can)
- 1/8 teaspoon ground allspice blend
- 1/4 teaspoon black pepper (ground)

Instructions:

1. Trim the fat from the meat and cut them into 1-inch pieces.
2. Place the chopped meat chunks into the slow cooker.
3. Add garlic, squash and onions to the contents in the cooker.
4. Pour the beef broth into the cooker.
5. Add the tomato sauce, dry mustard, garlic cloves, allspice blend and pepper to the cooker.
6. Cover the cooker and cook on high heat for 5 hours and in low heat setting for 10 hours

7. Take a small bowl and mix together the cornstarch and cold water. Ensure there are no lumps.
8. Pour this cornstarch mixture and green beans into the contents in the cooker.
9. Cover and cook for 15 minutes until the liquid thickens (if you have been cooking on low, change to high-heat setting).
10. Transfer to plate and serve warm.

Slow-Cooked Brisket in Onion Gravy

Makes: 14 servings

Carbs per serving: 8 grams

Ingredients:

- 5 pounds trimmed flat-cut beef brisket
- 4 finely sliced large onions
- 2 cups reduced-sodium beef broth
- 6 ounces tomato paste (1 can)
- 6 minced garlic cloves
- 2 tablespoons softened butter
- 2 tablespoons extra-virgin olive oil, divided
- 1 tablespoon Worcestershire sauce
- 2 tablespoons all-purpose flour
- 1 teaspoon black pepper (coarsely ground)
- 1 teaspoon dried thyme
- 1 teaspoon salt

Instructions:

1. Cut the brisket into three pieces small enough to fit into the Dutch oven.
2. Heat 1-tablespoon olive oil over medium-high heat in the Dutch oven.
3. Add one brisket piece to the hot oil and reduce the heat to medium.
4. Cook for 2 minutes until the brisket browns and flip over. Brown for 2 more minutes.
5. Repeat with the remaining brisket pieces and transfer the browned brisket to a slow cooker (*you can add the remaining oil if the meat gets sticky while you brown them*)

6. Cook the onions in the same Dutch oven (adding more oil if necessary) for 6 minutes until translucent.
7. Add the pepper, garlic and thyme to the Dutch oven and stir-fry for 1 minute.
8. Add the tomato paste, beef broth and salt to the mixture. Stir once until well combined.
9. Bring the contents to boil and transfer this onion-broth mixture to the slow cooker.
10. Cover the cooker and cook on high for 5 hours or on low heat for 10 hours until the brisket becomes tender and soft.
11. After the cooking cycle, remove the brisket from the cooker and place it on a cutting board.
12. Using 2 forks shred the briskets and transfer to a serving dish. Cover it with a foil to keep it warm.
13. Heat a saucepan over medium-high heat and pour the gravy from the cooker to the hot pan.
14. Bring it to boil and let it continue for 5 minutes until the gravy reduces.
15. Mix the flour and butter in a small bowl until you get a creamy smooth texture.
16. Lower the heat once the gravy reduces and let it simmer. Keep stirring as you continue to cook for 3 minutes until the liquid thickens.
17. Add the Worcestershire sauce and half the butter-flour mixture into the gravy. Mix it well and let simmer for 3 minutes.
18. If the gravy doesn't thicken to a creamy soup consistency, add the remaining butter mixture and simmer.

19. Once done, pour the gravy over the brisket and serve hot. Enjoy!

Slow Cooker Low Carb

Arianna Brooks

French Country Beef Stew

Makes: 8 servings

Carbs per serving: 8 grams

Ingredients:

- 3 1/2 pounds trimmed beef shank (sliced)
- 3 cups reduced-sodium beef broth
- 4 coarsely chopped turkey bacon slices
- 1 1/2 cups diced carrots, (2 medium ones should do)
- 2 cups dry red wine, such as Zinfandel or Merlot
- 1 1/2 cups finely chopped onion (2 medium ones)
- 2 bay leaves
- 2 orange zest (2 1/2-inch-long strips)
- 1/2 cup chopped parsley
- 1 teaspoon thyme leaves or 1/2 teaspoon dried thyme
- 1/2 cup diced celery (1 stalk should be enough)
- 2 teaspoons extra-virgin olive oil
- Freshly ground pepper, to taste
- Nonstick cooking spray

Instructions:

1. Heat oil in a medium-sized pot over medium-high heat. Add bacon to the hot oil and stir-fry for 5 minutes until lightly browned on all the sides.
2. Add onions, celery and carrots to the pot. Continue to cook for 10 minutes, stirring often, until the vegetables are lightly browned and softened.
3. Add the orange zest, thyme, bay leaves, broth and wine to the contents in the pot. Stir well and bring it to boil.

4. Rinse the beef thoroughly with cool water and remove if there are any bits of bone in it.
5. Lightly grease the inside of the slow cooker with a nonstick cooking spray and place the rinsed beef in it.
6. Turn on the heat and set it high. Pour the cooked vegetable mixture carefully from the pot over the beef in the cooker.
7. Cover the cooker and cook for 7 hours until the meat is tender enough to shred when pricked with a fork.
8. Once the cooking cycle is over, transfer the cooked beef from the cooker to a large bowl using a slotted spoon.
9. Remove the bones from the meat and discard. Break the meat with a spoon into small easy-to-bite chunks. Cover with an aluminum foil and set aside.
10. Remove the orange zest and the bay leaves from the sauce in the cooker. Skim out all the fat that is floating on the surface.
11. Take a large skillet and pour the entire sauce into it from the cooker. Heat the skillet over medium-high and bring the contents to boil.
12. Skim the froth as the liquid boils and let it continue for 20 minutes.
13. This will thicken the sauce and intensify the flavor. Sprinkle pepper and mix well.
14. Add the cooked boneless meat to the sauce and heat it through.
15. Transfer the stew into bowls and sprinkle the parsley over it.
16. Serve hot and enjoy!

Arianna Brooks

Fragrant Shredded Beef Stew

Makes: 10 servings

Carbs per serving: 15 grams

Ingredients:

- 3 pounds fat-trimmed flank steak (each steak cut into thirds)
- 1 seeded and chopped red bell pepper (large pepper)
- 1 1/2 cups reduced-sodium chicken broth
- 3 minced garlic cloves
- 2 finely sliced celery stalks
- 1 chopped large onion,
- 1/2 teaspoon pepper (freshly ground)
- 1 tablespoon ground cumin
- 1/2 cup pickled jalapenos (chopped)
- 1/4 cup sherry vinegar
- 10 heated corn tortillas
- 1 teaspoon salt
- 1/2 cup chopped fresh cilantro leaves (packed)

Instructions:

1. Pour the chicken broth in a slow cooker and add the garlic, celery, onion, bell pepper, cumin, pepper and salt to it.
2. Add the meat and ensure it is submerged in the liquid. Tuck the vegetables between, over and under the pieces.
3. Cover the cooker and cook on low heat for 8 hours or on high for 4 hours until the meat is soft and tender.
4. Once the cooking cycle is done, transfer the meat to a cutting board and let it sit for 10 minutes.

5. Using 2 forks shred the meat and place it back into the cooker.
6. Add the cilantro leaves and stir well.
7. To heat the corn tortillas, wrap them in a foil and bake at 300 degrees F for 10 minutes until it steams
8. Transfer the stew into a bowl and garnish with jalapeno.
9. Serve with the warm tortillas and enjoy!

Arianna Brooks

Coffee-Braised Pot Roast with Caramelized Onions

Makes: 10 servings

Carbs per serving: 4 grams

Ingredients:

- 3/4 cup brewed coffee (strong)
- 4 pounds fat-trimmed beef chuck roast
- 4 cups finely sliced onions (2 large ones)
- 2 tablespoons balsamic vinegar
- 4 minced garlic cloves
- 2 tablespoons cornstarch mixed with 2 tablespoons water
- 1 teaspoon dried thyme
- 4 teaspoons extra-virgin olive oil, divided
- 1/2 teaspoon salt
- Freshly ground pepper, to taste

Instructions:

1. Season the meat with pepper and salt. Keep aside.
2. Heat 2 teaspoons oil over medium-high heat in a pot and add the seasoned beef to the hot oil.
3. Cook for 7 minutes until browned on side. Turn over the meat often to ensure it doesn't get burnt.
4. Transfer the browned beef to the slow cooker.
5. Add the remaining oil to the cooker and throw in the thyme and garlic to it.
6. Pour 1/2 cup strongly brewed coffee to the contents in the cooker and mix well.

7. Add vinegar, cover the cooker and cook on high for 5 hours or on low for 8 hours.
8. Once the cooking cycle is over, transfer the cooked meat to a cutting board and slice them into chunks.
9. Heat a pot over medium-high heat and pour the liquid from the cooker into it.
10. Bring it to boil and skim off the fat from the surface of the liquid. Add the cornstarch mixture and continue to cook.
11. Whisk the liquid carefully for 60 seconds until it thickens. Transfer the meat chunks back into the liquid and season with pepper if desired.
12. Serve hot and enjoy!

Arianna Brooks

Texas Beef and Beans

Makes: 8 servings

Carbs per serving: 15 grams

Ingredients:

- 3 pounds boneless arm chuck roast
- 15 ounces drained and rinsed pinto beans (1 can)
- 1 medium onion (cut into wedges)
- 1/3 cup chipotle barbecue sauce
- 14 1/2 ounces diced tomatoes (1 can), drained
- 1 4 ounces diced green chilies (1 can)
- 1 teaspoon crushed dried oregano
- 1 teaspoon ground cumin
- 2 teaspoons chili powder
- 1/2 teaspoon garlic powder

Instructions:

1. Trim the fat from the chuck roast and place it in a slow cooker.
2. Add garlic powder, chili powder, cumin and oregano to the meat. Season it well.
3. Add the green chilies, tomatoes, onions and beans over the seasoned meat.
4. Cover the cooker and cook on high for 5 hours or on low heat for 10 hours
5. Once the cooking cycle is over, remove the roast and cut it into 8 portions.
6. Put it back into the mixture in the cooker. Add the barbeque sauce and stir well.

7. Cover the cooker and cook on high for 5 minutes until the contents are heated through.

Slow Cooker Ham and Egg Casserole

Makes: 4 servings

Carbs per serving: 2.5 grams

Ingredients:

- 1 pound trimmed ham steak (chopped into cubes)
- 6 eggs
- 1 cup shredded cheese
- 1/2 cup heavy cream
- 1 tablespoon butter (melted)
- 2 finely chopped green onions
- Black pepper, to taste
- Nonstick cooking spray

Instructions:

1. Grease the insides of the slow cooker bowl with a nonstick cooking spray and add the melted butter.
2. Place the chopped ham and green onions in the cooker bowl.
3. Take a large bowl and crack the eggs. Beat the eggs thoroughly until combined.
4. Add the cream and whisk the contents until smooth.
5. Pour this into the slow cooker and add the pepper. Mix well.
6. Add the cheese and mix for one last time.
7. Close the cooker and cook on high for an hour. Stir in between to ensure the contents are cooked evenly.

8. Once the cooking cycle is over, stir the entire contents thoroughly. Close the lid and cook on high for additional 30 minutes
9. When the center part is nicely cooked, transfer to a plate and serve hot.

Low Carb Chili

Makes: 4 servings

Carbs per serving: 10 grams

Ingredients:

- 1 pound ground beef
- 1 deseeded and chopped red bell pepper
- 1 pound ground pork
- 1 teaspoon onion powder
- 2 teaspoons garlic paste
- 1 teaspoon paprika
- 15 ounces passata tomato sauce (1 can)
- 1 tablespoon Worcestershire Sauce
- 1 teaspoon ground cumin
- Nonstick cooking spray
- Shredded cheese, for garnishing

Instructions:

1. Grease a large skillet with nonstick cooking spray.
2. Preheat the skillet over medium heat and add the pork to the hot skillet.
3. Add garlic and beef along with the pork. Cook until the meat has thoroughly browned.
4. Drain the fat and transfer the meat to the slow cooker.
5. Add the onion powder, garlic paste, paprika, tomato sauce, Worcestershire sauce and cumin to the cooker.
6. Mix well until the ingredients are combined completely.
7. Cover the cooker and cook on high for 3 hours.
8. If you are cooking on low heat, cook for 6 hours.

9. Transfer to a plate and serve with shredded cheese. Enjoy!

Simple Pepper Steak

Makes: 3 servings

Carbs per serving: 15 grams

Ingredients:

- 3/4 lb. beef round steak, sliced into strips
- 1/8 cup and 1/2 Tbsp. flour, divided
- 1/8 tsp pepper
- 1/2 cup sliced onion
- 1/4 tsp minced garlic
- 3/4 cup sliced green pepper
- 14 oz. unsalted diced tomatoes
- 1/2 Tbsp. unsalted soy sauce
- 1/2 tsp Worcestershire sauce
- 1 1/2 Tbsp. water

Instructions:

1. In a small bowl, mix together the pepper and flour 1/8-cup flour.
2. Place the beef strips in the slow cooker and toss the flour and pepper mixture until all the pieces are well coated.
3. Sprinkle the garlic, green pepper, and onions into the slow cooker and combine with the beef.
4. In a bowl, mix together the diced tomato, Worcestershire sauce and soy sauce, then pour the mixture into the slow cooker and mix all of the ingredients well.
5. Cover and cook for 8 hours on low. Mix together the remaining flour with the water until you have a paste. Stir this mixture into the slow cooker. Cover and cook

until the sauce becomes thick. Serve with cauliflower rice or cooked quinoa.

Easy Italian Steak

Makes: 3 servings

Carbs per serving: 14 grams

Ingredients:

- 3/4 lb. beef round steak, sliced into 3 equal portions
- 1/4 tsp oregano
- 1/8 tsp pepper
- 1/2 cup coarsely chopped onion
- 7 1/2 oz. low sodium spaghetti sauce

Instructions:

1. In a mixing bowl, combine the pepper and oregano. Rub this mixture all over each slice of beef, then put the beef into the slow cooker.
2. Put the chopped onion on top of the beef, then add the spaghetti sauce carefully. Cover and cook for 5 hours on low, or until the beef is well done.

Arianna Brooks

Beer-braised Short Ribs

Makes: 4 servings

Carbs per serving: 10 grams

Ingredients:

- 1 1/2 lb. beef short ribs
- 1 Tbsp. packed brown sugar
- 1/2 tsp minced garlic
- 1/2 cup chopped onion
- 1/2 cup low sodium beef broth
- 1/8 cup flour
- 6 oz. beer (dark or ale)

Instructions:

1. Put the beef into the slow cooker, then mix in the flour, brown sugar, and garlic. Coat each piece very well. Sprinkle the onions on top of the beef.
2. In a small bowl, combine the beer and broth, then pour this mixture into the slow cooker.
3. Cover and cook for 8 hours on low, or until the beef becomes very tender.

Barbecue Brisket

Makes: 5 servings

Carbs per serving: 8 grams

Ingredients:

- 2 lb. beef brisket
- 4 oz. unsalted tomato sauce
- 6 oz. beer
- 1 tsp prepared mustard
- 1 Tbsp. Worcestershire sauce
- 1 Tbsp. balsamic vinegar
- 1/2 tsp garlic powder
- 1/8 tsp pepper
- 1/4 tsp ground allspice
- 1/2 Tbsp. brown sugar
- 1/2 cup chopped red bell pepper
- 1/2 cup chopped onion

Instructions:

1. Put the beef brisket into the slow cooker.
2. In a bowl, mix together all of the other ingredients, then pour this mixture on top of the beef brisket, coating the meat very well.
3. Cover and cook for 8 hours on low, then take out the beef brisket from the sauce and shred very well. Put the shredded meat back into the slow cooker and mix it with the sauce, then serve.

Arianna Brooks

Beef Roast with Apples

Makes: 4 to 5 servings

Carbs per serving: 5 grams

Ingredients:

- 1 1/2 lb. beef round roast
- 1/2 cup water
- 1/4 tsp Worcestershire sauce
- 1/8 tsp garlic powder
- 1 apple, quartered
- 1/2 cup sliced onion
- A dash each of: chili powder, celery seed, nutmeg, coriander, onion powder, paprika, garlic powder, turmeric

Instructions:

1. Place a greased non-stick skillet over medium flame and cook the beef until browned on all sides. Place into the slow cooker.
2. Pour the water into the same skillet and gently scrape off any browned bits, then pour this into the slow cooker as well.
3. Sprinkle the seasonings into the slow cooker, then add the Worcestershire sauce, apple pieces, and sliced onion.
4. Cover and cook for 5 hours on low, or until the meat becomes very tender.

Sour Cream Pot Roast

Makes: 4 servings

Carbs per serving: 5 grams

Ingredients:

- 2 lb. beef chuck roast
- 1/2 clove garlic
- 1/4 tsp pepper
- 1/4 cup sliced onion
- 1/4 cup chopped celery
- 1/4 cup chopped carrot
- 1/3 cup sour cream
- 1 1/2 Tbsp. flour
- 1/4 cup dry white wine

Instructions:

1. Rub the garlic clove all over the roast, then season with the pepper. Place the roast into the slow cooker. Add the carrots, onion, and celery in with them.
2. Mix together the wine, sour cream, and flour, then pour the mixture into the slow cooker. Cover and cook for 6 hours on low.

Arianna Brooks

Mexican Steak Stew

Makes: 4 servings

Carbs per serving: 5 grams

Ingredients:

- 1 1/4 lb. beef round roast, excess fat trimmed off
- 1/2 cup chopped onion
- 7 oz. unsalted diced tomatoes, undrained
- 1/2 cup sliced red bell pepper
- A dash each of: ground dried chili peppers, garlic powder, onion powder, paprika, cumin, celery seed, oregano, cayenne, and ground bay leaf

Instructions:

1. Slice the beef into 2 inch pieces, then place them into the slow cooker and stir in the onion.
2. In a bowl, combine the seasonings with the undrained diced tomatoes and pour this mixture on top of the beef. Sprinkle the red pepper on top.
3. Cover and cook for 6 hours on low or until the beef becomes very tender.

Beef with Eggplant

Makes: 3 servings

Carbs per serving: 6 grams

Ingredients:

- 1 cup peeled and cubed eggplant,
- 4 oz. unsalted tomato sauce
- 1/4 cup chopped celery
- 1/4 cup chopped green pepper
- 1/4 cup chopped onion
- 1/8 tsp nutmeg
- 1/8 tsp crushed marjoram
- 1/8 tsp cinnamon
- 3/4 lb. beef round steak, sliced into small cubes

Instructions:

1. Combine the eggplant, onion, celery, green pepper, tomato sauce, cinnamon, nutmeg, and marjoram in the slow cooker.
2. Place the cubed beef on top of everything, then cover and cook for 8 hours on low.

Arianna Brooks

Beef Osso Buco

Makes: 5 servings

Carbs per serving: 10.8 grams

Ingredients:

- 1 ½ pounds cross-cut bone-in beef shanks
- 1 teaspoon kosher salt, divided or to taste
- 2 teaspoons canola oil, divided
- Cooking spray
- 1 cup onions, sliced
- ½ cup carrots, chopped
- ½ cup celery, chopped
- 1 tablespoon tomato paste
- 4 cloves garlic, crushed
- ½ cup beef stock, unsalted
- ¼ ounce dried porcini mushrooms, chopped
- ¼ cup red wine
- 1 teaspoon corn starch
- Black pepper powder to taste
- 1 bay leaf
- 4 plum tomatoes
- 3 tablespoons fresh flat leaf parsley
- ½ tablespoon lemon rind, grated
- ½ tablespoon garlic, minced
- Salt to taste

Instructions:

1. Season the beef shank with half the salt. Spray the pot of the slow cooker with cooking spray.

2. Preheat a broiler. Broil the tomatoes until they are blackish. Crush the tomatoes lightly.
3. Place a skillet over medium heat. Add 1-teaspoon oil. Add the beef and cook on both the sides until browned. Transfer the beef to the pot.
4. To the same skillet, add a teaspoon of oil. Add onion, celery, crushed garlic, and carrot. Sauté for a minute. Add tomato paste and sauté for 3-4 minutes. Add mushroom and stock. Stir well and pour into the cooker after scraping the pan to remove the browned bits. Add wine, cornstarch, pepper and bay leaf. Mix well.
5. Place the blackened tomatoes over the beef.
6. Cover and cook on low for 8 hours or until done. When done, remove the beef from the pot. Remove and discard the bones and the bay leaf and put the meat back to the pot.
7. Sprinkle minced garlic, lemon rind, and parsley and serve.

Arianna Brooks

Mexican Beef

Makes: 12 servings

Carbs per serving: 1.9 grams

Ingredients:

- 3 lbs. of boneless beef chuck (shoulder roast)
- 1 tbsp. of ground coriander
- 1 tbsp. of ground cumin
- 1 tbsp. of chili powder
- ½ tsp of ground red pepper
- 1 tsp of salt
- 1 cup of salsa
- 1 tbsp. of corn starch
- 2 tbsp. of water

Instructions:

1. Cut beef chuck in half and place it inside the slow cooker.
2. In a small mixing bowl, combine the coriander, cumin, salt, chili powder and red pepper then rub the mixture on the roast.
3. Place ½ cup of the salsa into the slow cooker and place beef roast on top. Then, add in the remaining salsa and cover.
4. Cook for 10 hours on low setting. Once done, remove the roast from the slow cooker and let it cool slightly. Remove the excess fat from the beef and shred using a fork.

5. Remove the excess fat on top of the cooking liquid then combine the water and cornstarch until it becomes smooth.
6. Pour it into the slow cooker and whisk to combine. Cook for 15 minutes on high settings.
7. Return the beef into the slow cooker and cover. Cook for another 15 minutes then adjust the seasoning before serving.

Arianna Brooks

Beef Pot Roast with Mushrooms

Makes: 3 servings

Carbs per serving: 7.4 grams

Ingredients:

- 4 ounce package pre sliced mushroom,
- 1 pound boneless shoulder pot roast
- 4 ounce green bell pepper, refrigerated, pre chopped
- Cooking spray
- 3 tablespoons ketchup
- ¼ teaspoon black pepper powder
- Salt to taste

Instructions:

1. Mix together in a small bowl, ketchup, salt, and pepper.
2. Place a skillet over medium heat. Spray the skillet cooking spray. Add the roast and cook until browned on both the sides.
3. Spray the pot of the slow cooker with cooking spray.
4. Place the mushrooms and bell pepper at the bottom of the pot.
5. Place the browned pot roast over the mushrooms. Pour the ketchup mixture over the roast.
6. Cover and cook on high for an hour and then low for 7 hours or until the roast is done.
7. To serve, place the mushrooms and bell pepper over the roast.

Spicy Braised Beef

Makes: 3 servings

Carbs per serving: 5.3 grams

Ingredients:

- 1 pound lean beef top round, trimmed of fat
- 1 small onion, diced
- 1 small red bell pepper, diced
- 2 cloves garlic, sliced
- 2 spicy peppers of your choice, chopped
- ¼ cup low sodium beef broth
- ½ cup canned, diced tomatoes with juice
- ½ tablespoon Worcestershire sauce
- 1 tablespoon fresh lime juice
- ½ teaspoon cumin powder
- ¼ teaspoon dried oregano
- ¼ teaspoon dried coriander

Instructions:

1. Mix together in a bowl beef broth, Worcestershire sauce, tomatoes, lime juice, oregano, cumin and coriander.
2. Place the beef in the slow cooker. Sprinkle salt and pepper. Pour the sauce mixture over the beef. Sprinkle the onion, pepper, garlic, and red pepper all over and around the beef.
3. Cover and cook on a low flame for 8 hours. After about 7 ½ hours, cut the beef into strips and cook for the remaining 30 minutes.
4. Serve hot.

Arianna Brooks

Puerto Rican Beef Encebollado

Makes: 3 servings

Carbs per serving: 7 grams

Ingredients:

- 1 pound lean beef roast
- 2 onions, thinly sliced
- ½ cup beef broth
- 2 tablespoons white vinegar
- ½ teaspoon dried oregano
- Salt to taste
- Pepper powder to taste

Instructions:

1. Mix together in a bowl the broth, vinegar, and oregano.
2. Place the beef in the pot of the slow cooker. Sprinkle salt and pepper.
3. Cover the beef with onions and garlic.
4. Pour the broth mixture over the onions.
5. Cover and cook on low for about 8 hours or until done.

Traditional Ropa Vieja

Makes: 8 servings

Carbs per serving: 14 grams

Ingredients:

- 2 lbs. of beef skirt steak
- 14 oz. of beef broth
- 1 tbsp. of cooking oil
- 8 oz. of tomato sauce
- 1 tbsp. of red wine vinegar
- 6 oz. of tomato paste
- 1 small onion, sliced into thin strips
- 2 cloves of garlic, minced
- 1 green bell pepper, sliced into thin strips
- 1 tsp of cumin
- 1 tsp of red pepper flakes

Instructions:

1. Prepare a large pan and set it over medium to high heat. Add in the cooking oil. Once the oil is hot, add in the beef and cook until all sides are browned equally. Remove the meat from the pan and set it aside.
2. Add in the beef broth, tomato sauce, and tomato paste, red wine vinegar, onion, green bell pepper, garlic cloves, cumin and red pepper flakes into the pan. Stir until well combined and make sure to get the browned bits off from the bottom of the pan.
3. Pour the contents of the pan into the slow cooker and place the beef on top. Spoon the mixture over the beef to coat the meat lightly.
4. Cover and cook for 9 hours on low setting.

Arianna Brooks

Hearty Beef Stew

Makes: 16 servings

Carbs per serving: 3.5 grams

Ingredients:

- 1 tsp. of dried oregano
- 1 tsp. of onion powder
- 1 tsp. of garlic powder
- 1 ½ tsp. of black pepper
- 2 tsp. of sea salt
- 2 tbsp. of Worcestershire sauce
- 2 tbsp. of organic tomato paste
- 4 cloves of garlic (large), minced
- 1 onion (small), chopped
- 1 carrot (large), chopped
- 2 ribs of celery, chopped
- 4oz of mushrooms, quartered
- 4oz of mixed bell peppers, chopped
- 14.5oz of organic diced tomatoes, drained
- 12oz of bacon, cooked crisp then crumbled
- 2 cups of organic beef stock
- 3 tbsp. of olive oil
- 2lbs of stew beef

Instructions:

1. Preheat the slow cooker by turning it on and setting it on low heat.
2. In a pan placed over medium heat, add in the olive oil and sear the stew beef until both sides are browned well. Then, transfer the meat into the slow cooker.

3. Add in the dried oregano, onion powder, garlic powder, black pepper, sea salt, Worcestershire sauce, tomato paste, garlic, onion, carrot, celery, mushrooms, bell peppers, tomatoes, bacon, and beef stock to the slow cooker.
4. Cover and cook for 8 hours on low settings.

Stuffed Peppers

Makes: 1 serving

Carbs per serving: 7 grams

Ingredients:

- 3 tbsp. of tomato sauce
- 1 tbsp. of chopped onion
- 1/3lb of ground beef
- 1/3 cup of finely chopped cauliflower
- 1 Poblano pepper

Instructions:

1. Halve the Poblano pepper lengthwise and remove the seeds. Set it aside.
2. In a pan, brown the onion and ground beef. Add in the tomato sauce and cauliflower and stir. Then, spoon the mixture into the pepper halves.
3. Add in about ½ inch of tomato juice or water into the slow cooker and lay the peppers carefully on top.
4. Cover and cook for 4 hours on low settings.

Arianna Brooks

Kicking Chili

Makes: 16 servings

Carbs per serving: 4.7 grams

Ingredients:

- 1 bay leaf
- 1 tsp. of black pepper
- 1 tsp. of oregano
- 1 tsp. of onion powder
- 1 tsp. of garlic powder
- ½ tsp. of cayenne
- 2 tsp. of salt
- 2 ½ tbsp. of cumin, mounded
- 4 tbsp. of chili powder
- 2 tbsp. of Worcestershire sauce
- 14.5oz of stewed tomatoes (with Mexican seasoning)
- 14.5oz of tomatoes with green chilies
- 6oz of tomato paste
- ¼ cup of jalapeno slices
- 3 ribs of celery (large), diced
- 4 tbsp. of minced garlic
- 1 red onion (medium), chopped
- 2 ½lbs of lean ground beef

Instructions:

1. Preheat the slow cooker using low settings.
2. In a pan placed on medium-high heat, add in 2 tablespoons of the minced garlic, half of the onion, ground beef, pepper, and salt. Cook until the beef is brown in color. Remove the excess grease.

3. Transfer the contents of the pan into the slow cooker. Add in the bay leaf, black pepper, oregano, onion powder, garlic powder, cayenne, salt, cumin, chili powder, Worcestershire sauce, stewed tomatoes, tomatoes and green chilies, tomato paste, jalapenos, celery, garlic, and the remaining onion.
4. Stir the ingredients together until properly combined. Cover and cook for 8 hours on low settings.

Arianna Brooks

Beef Rags

Makes: 6 servings

Carbs per serving: 3 grams

Ingredients:

- 3 tbsp. of olive oil (unfiltered and extra-virgin)
- ½ tbsp. of Dijon mustard
- 1 cup of cabernet sauvignon
- 2 tbsp. of Worcestershire sauce
- ½ tbsp. of black pepper (freshly ground)
- ½ tbsp. of kosher salt
- 1 tsp. of onion powder
- 2 tsp. of granulated garlic
- 3lbs of chuck roast

Instructions:

1. Season the chuck roast using the kosher salt, black pepper, granulated garlic, and onion powder. Place the seasoned meat in a Dutch oven with ½ of the olive oil and set it on medium-high heat. Sear the chuck roast for 4 minutes on each side. About halfway through searing, add in the remaining olive oil into the Dutch oven.
2. Once the meat is browned, transfer it into the slow cooker and slather with Worcestershire sauce and Dijon mustard. Pour in the dry red wine and cover. Cook for 8 hours or until the meat becomes very tender.
3. Once cooking time is done, separate the chuck roast and pass the sauce through a strainer to remove any

bone or stringy fat. Break up the meat into rags using a fork, and stir it into the strained sauce.

Arianna Brooks

Swiss Steak

Makes: 6 servings

Carbs per serving: 4 grams

Ingredients:

- 2 cloves of garlic (peeled and minced)
- ½ cup of bell pepper
- ½ cup of sliced carrots
- ½ cup of sliced onions
- 1 cup of sliced celery
- 1 1/3 cups of beef broth
- 1 tbsp. of liquid smoke (mesquite flavor)
- 14.5oz of tomatoes
- 2 ½lbs of round steak (boneless)
- ½ tsp. of kosher salt
- Freshly ground pepper

Instructions:

1. Add in the garlic, bell pepper, carrots, onions, celery, beef broth, liquid smoke, tomatoes, steak, kosher salt and pepper into the slow cooker. Give it a stir and make sure that the meat is well coated with the sauce.
2. Cook and cover for 10 hours on low settings.

Coffee Brisket

Makes: 8 servings

Carbs per serving: 8 grams

Ingredients:

- 1 tbsp. of balsamic vinegar
- ½ cup of strong brewed coffee
- 2 onion (large), sliced
- 3lbs of beef brisket (boneless)
- 1 tsp. of salt
- 1 tsp. of ground black pepper
- 1 tsp. of garlic powder
- 1 tbsp. of paprika
- 1 tbsp. of ground coffee
- 2 tbsp. of brown sugar

Instructions:

1. In a mixing bowl, combine the salt, pepper, garlic powder, paprika, ground coffee, and brown sugar. Trim the excess fat from the brisket and rub the spice mixture on all the surfaces of the beef.
2. Place the meat inside the slow cooker. Cut the meat, if necessary. Place the onions on top of the beef. Combine the vinegar and coffee and pour it over the onions.
3. Cover and cook for 10 hours on low settings or 5 hours on high settings. Transfer the meat on a cutting board and slice it across the grain. Remove the onions from the slow cooker using a slotted spoon and place it on the meat. Serve.

Arianna Brooks

Beef and Beans

Makes: 8 servings

Carbs per serving: 15g

Ingredients:

- 1/3 cup of chipotle barbecue sauce
- 4oz of diced green chilies
- 14.5oz can of diced tomatoes, drained
- 15oz can of pinto beans, drained then rinsed
- 1 onion (medium), cut into wedges
- ½ tsp. of garlic powder
- 1 tsp. of dried oregano, crushed
- 1 tsp. of ground cumin
- 2 tsp. of chili powder
- 3lbs of arm chuck roast (boneless)

Instructions:

1. Trim the excess fat from the chuck roast and place it inside the slow cooker. Use the garlic powder, oregano, cumin, and chili powder to season the meat. Then, place the green chilies, tomatoes, beans, and onion on top. Cover and cook for 10 hours on low settings or 5 hours on high.
2. Once done, remove the roast and divide it into 8 equal portions. Then, adjust the slow cooker to high heat and stir the barbecue sauce. Replace the roast into the slow cooker and stir and cook for another 5 minutes.

Beef Stroganoff

Makes: 4 servings

Carbs per serving: 7.2 grams

Ingredients:

- 1 ¼ pound beef eye of round or bottom round roast, trimmed of fat
- 1 medium onion, diced
- 2 cloves garlic, minced
- 6 ounce whole baby mushrooms of your choice
- 1 tablespoon Worcestershire sauce
- ¾ tablespoon whole grain mustard
- ¾ tablespoon balsamic vinegar
- ¾ cup beef broth
- ½ tablespoon arrowroot
- 1 bay leaf
- ¼ cup low fat sour cream
- 2 tablespoon low fat cream cheese
- 1 teaspoon fresh thyme

Instructions:

1. Sprinkle the beef with salt and pepper.
2. Mix together in a bowl Worcestershire sauce, vinegar, mustard, broth, and arrowroot.
3. Place the beef in the pot of the slow cooker. Add onions, garlic, bay leaf, and mushrooms.
4. Pour the sauce over and around the beef.
5. Cover and cook on low for 8 hours.
6. During the last 15 minutes of the cooking process, add sour cream, cream cheese, and thyme.
7. When done, discard the bay leaf.

Arianna Brooks

Autumn Oxtail Stew

Makes: 4 servings

Carbs per serving: 5.8 grams

Ingredients:

- 2 kg oxtail or beef suitable for slow-cooking, yields approximately 50% meat
- 1 tbsp. ghee, lard or butter
- 2 cups beef stock, water, or vegetable stock
- 1 carrot
- 1 red onion
- 1 garlic head
- 2 stalks celery
- Peel and juice from 1 average-sized orange
- 5-8 cloves
- 1 cinnamon stick
- 1/4 tsp nutmeg
- 1 star anise
- 2 bay leaves (dried or fresh)
- Black pepper, freshly ground to taste
- 1/2 tsp salt to taste
- 2 heads medium lettuce or 4 heads small lettuce

Instructions:

1. Pre-heat oven to 300º F/150º C. Season meat with some salt & pepper.
2. Put the oxtail in a large pre-heated non-stick pan previously greased w/ ghee. Brown on each side briefly.
3. Transfer the meat to a baking dish.

4. Get the large red onion; peel and halve. Take the orange and juice. Halve the garlic head. Peel the carrot.
5. Put all the spices into a pot, boil and cook for around 5 minutes. Afterwards, remove from the heat, and set it aside.
6. Get all ingredients from the pot, and place on top of the oxtail (browned). Cook for 3 to 4 hours until the meat is tender or almost falls apart.
7. Once done, take the dish out of the oven and allow to cool down. Remove all spices, veggies, and orange (the softened veggies are edible).
8. Get a fork to separate the bones from the meat. Place the meat in a bowl and pour enough sauce over it.
9. Fold shredded meat on fresh leaves of lettuce. Serve and enjoy!

Corned Beef & Cabbage

Makes: 3 to 4 servings

Carbs per serving: 4 grams

Ingredients:

- 1 pc corned beef brisket (3 to 4 lbs.)
- 12 oz. beef broth or beer
- 1 beef bouillon
- 1 tsp allspice
- 1 tsp ground pepper
- 3 cloves garlic, crushed
- 1 small-sized green cabbage head, divided in 8 thick wedges w/out the core and outer leaves

Instructions:

1. Get the corned beef brisket and rinse it with water thoroughly.
2. Place the beef with all other ingredients into the slow cooker, except for the cabbage. Allow to cook for 6 hours on low heat.
3. Mix the cabbage wedges in, and cook for an additional hour, still on low heat setting.
4. After cooking, trim excess fat off.
5. Serve with horseradish sauce or whole grain mustard. If desired, season the cabbage.

Arianna Brooks

Tri-Tip Tacos

Makes: 8 servings

Carbs per serving: 1.1 grams

Ingredients:

- 1 tbsp. of ancho chili powder
- 1 tbsp. of smoked paprika
- 8 cloves of garlic
- 2 lbs. of lean tri-tip sirloin, roasted and fat trimmed
- 1 pc onion, chopped
- 1 cup beef broth
- 1 bay leaf
- 1 tsp. black pepper
- 1 tsp. salt

Instructions:

1. First, you have to turn garlic into paste form. To do this, you can use a food processor to pulse it, or use a garlic press. You can also mince it and press it until it becomes paste-like using a pinch of coarse salt and the backside of your knife.
2. Combine the chili powder, paprika, and salt & pepper with the garlic paste to produce a rub. Use the rub to cover the tri-tip sirloin roast (or grilled, depending on your preference.)
3. Add the onions and the beef broth in the slow cooker. Put the tri-tip at the top. Allow to cook for about 8 hours on low heat setting. 30 minutes before cooking time ends, take the lid off, then shred the pork meat.

Leave the cooker uncovered, and allow to cook for another 30 minutes.
4. Serve over rice, in warm corn tortillas, in lettuce wrap, or wrapped as burritos.

Arianna Brooks

Ropa Vieja Variation

Makes: 6 servings

Carbs per serving: 5.2 grams

Ingredients:

- 1.5 lbs. of flank steak, fat trimmed
- 1 yellow pepper
- 1 green pepper
- 1 onion, thinly sliced
- 3 or 4 cloves garlic, minced
- 1 bay leaf
- 3/4 tsp oregano
- 3/4 tsp cumin
- 3/4 cup chicken or beef broth
- 3 tbsp. of tomato paste
- 1/3 tsp. salt
- 3 tbsp. green olives, sliced; or 1 tbsp. of capers (optional)

Instructions:

1. Spray the crockpot with some cooking spray. If preferred, you can use a crockpot liner.
2. Combine all the ingredients in the crockpot, and stir well.
3. Allow to cook on low heat setting for about 6 hours. Depending on the crockpot used, the cooking time may vary slightly.

Korean Beef Tacos

Makes: 10 servings

Carbs per serving: 6.5 grams

Ingredients:

- 2 lbs. beef roast, fat trimmed
- 10 cloves garlic, intact
- 1/2 cup of brown sugar
- 2 jalapenos, diced
- 1/3 cup of soy sauce
- 1/2 red onion, diced
- 1 inch ginger root, fresh, peeled & grated
- 2 tbsp. rice wine vinegar, seasoned
- 2 tbsp. sesame seeds

Instructions:

1. In a small-sized bowl, mix the soy sauce, sugar, jalapenos, red onion, sesame seeds, and rice vinegar.
2. Put the beef and garlic inside the crockpot. Pour the sauce.
3. Allow to cook on low heat for about 8 to 10 hours. Half an hour before the end of your allotted cooking time, check to see if you can easily shred the beef using a fork. If so, break the meat into large pieces. Continue to cook uncovered to thicken up the sauce.
4. Shred the beef some more before serving with warm corn tortillas and jicama slaw.
5. *For the Jicama Slaw*
6. Mix ½ bag of coleslaw mix, ¼ chopped cilantro, ½ diced jicama, ¼ cup of diced red onions, 1 tsp of Asian hot sauce, 2 tbsp. of peanut dressing, and the juice of 2

pieces of lime. Combine well, then serve on top or on the side of the taco.

Beef Machaca

Makes: 12 servings

Carbs per serving: 3 grams

Ingredients:

- 3 lbs. beef brisket or lean rump, roasted, fat trimmed
- 1/2 cup of beef broth
- 2 tbsp. Worcestershire sauce or 2 tbsp. of Maggi sauce
- 1 1/2 cups onion, diced
- 1 cup of red bell pepper, diced
- 4 tbsp. of fresh lime juice
- 3 cloves garlic, minced
- 3 pcs serrano chili, stemmed, seeded, & minced
- Salt & pepper
- 1/2 tsp dried oregano
- 1/2 14 oz. can of diced tomatoes w/ juice

Instructions:

1. Season the meat with some salt & pepper. Put it inside the slow cooker.
2. Whisk the beef broth, lime juice, and seasoning together in a medium-sized bowl. Stir the other ingredients in, then pour the mixture over the meat.
3. Cook for around 8 hours on low heat setting. Using 2 forks shred the beef.
4. Immediately serve and enjoy.

Arianna Brooks

Italian Beef

Makes: 8 servings

Carbs per serving: 1.8 grams

Ingredients:

- 2 lb. beef brisket, boneless, all fat trimmed
- 1 tbsp. of dried Italian seasoning
- 1 onion, sliced
- 4 to 6 cloves garlic, minced
- 2 cups of fat free beef broth
- 1 tsp red pepper, flaked
- 1/2 cup red wine
- Salt & pepper

Instructions:

1. Season the brisket with salt & pepper.
2. Combine all the ingredients in the slow cooker. Allow 8 hours to cook on low heat setting or until the meat easily shreds using a fork. If you intend to use the beef for sandwiches, strain the broth to create a dipping.

Beef Ragu

Makes: 10 servings

Carbs per serving: 3.8 grams

Ingredients:

- 4 lbs. of lean beef chuck, fat trimmed
- 1 rib celery, diced
- 1/2 onion, diced
- 1 carrot, peeled & diced
- 1 14.5 oz. can of crushed tomatoes
- 1 14.5 oz. can of diced tomatoes
- 1 ½ cups of beef broth
- 4 cloves of garlic, minced
- 2 bay leaves
- 2 tbsp. of fresh rosemary, minced
- 2 tbsp. of fresh thyme or oregano, chopped
- Salt & pepper

Instructions:

1. Place the celery, carrots, garlic, and onion at the bottom of the crockpot.
2. Generously season the meat with salt & pepper then put it in the cooker.
3. Add the rest of the ingredients. Cook for 6 to 8 hours or until the beef shreds easily with a fork.
4. Serve preferably with polenta or pasta, or even as a sandwich.

Arianna Brooks

Shredded Asian Beef

Makes: 10 servings

Carbs per serving: 3.8 grams

Ingredients:

- 3 lbs. beef eye or bottom round, roasted, fat trimmed
- 1/4 cups of rice wine vinegar
- 1/4 cups of brown sugar
- 2 tbsp. of ketchup
- 1/2 cups of soy sauce
- 2 tbsp. of sesame seeds
- 1 inch ginger, grated or minced
- 1 to 3 tsp of Asian chili sauce (optional)
- 1/2 red onion, minced
- 8 cloves of garlic, whole
- 1 to 2 jalapenos, seeded & minced

Instructions:

1. Whisk together the vinegar, soy sauce, ketchup, brown sugar, ginger, sesame seeds, and hot sauce (if preferred) in a small-sized bowl.
2. Stir the garlic cloves, jalapenos, and the onion in.
3. Put the beef inside the slow cooker, then pour the sauce on top. Let it cook for around 8 hours or until the beef is tender enough to shred easily with a fork.
4. Finish shredding the beef, and let it stay in the cooker for an extra half an hour to allow all the juices to blend well.
5. Remove from the crockpot and transfer to a serving dish.

6. Serve immediately.

Thai Curry Ground Beef

Makes: 4 servings

Arianna Brooks

Carbs per serving: 8 grams

Ingredients:

- 1 lb. of ground beef, lean
- 1 medium-sized leek, thinly sliced
- 2 cloves garlic, minced
- 1/2 cup of light coconut milk
- 1 tsp. ginger, minced
- 1 ½ cups of tomato sauce
- 1 tsp. of lime zest
- 1 tsp. of red curry paste
- 1 tbsp. of soy sauce
- 2 tsp. of lime juice

Instructions:

1. Cook the ground beef until brown before adding to the slow cooker with the garlic, leek, red curry paste, ginger, soy sauce, tomato sauce, and lime zest.
2. Allow to cook for about 4 hours on low heat setting.
3. Remove the lid and add the lime juice and coconut milk. Stir a little. Cook for another 15 minutes before serving.
4. Enjoy!

Chapter Five - Main Course - Pork and Lamb

Pork Stroganoff

Makes: 3 servings

Carbs per serving: 8 grams

Ingredients:

- ¾ pound stew meat, cut into 1 ½ inch cubes
- ½ teaspoon chicken bouillon granules
- ½ cup onion, chopped
- ½ tablespoon cornstarch mixed with 1 tablespoon water
- 1 tablespoon fresh parsley, snipped
- ¾ cup water
- 1 teaspoon paprika
- 1 small clove garlic, minced
- 6 tablespoons sour cream
- 6 oz. noodles, cooked, drained
- Cooking spray

Instructions:

1. Place a pan over medium heat. Add pork and cook until brown. Turn off the heat. Drain the fat in the pan.
2. Add water, paprika, bouillon, onion and garlic into the slow cooker and stir.
3. Place pork and stir.
4. Cover the pot and cook on Low for 6 to 7 hours or on High for 3 to 4 hours.

5. Add cornstarch mixture during the last 30 minutes of cooking. Stir frequently until the mixture thickens.
6. Add sour cream and parsley and mix well.
7. Divide the noodles into bowls. Top with pork and serve.

Pork Paprikash

Makes: 4 servings

Carbs per serving: 6 grams

Ingredients:

- 1 ¼ pounds lean pork tenderloin
- 2 cloves garlic, minced
- ½ tablespoon paprika
- ½ tablespoon Worcestershire sauce
- 2 tablespoons chicken broth
- A handful fresh thyme, chopped
- ¼ cup light sour cream
- ½ cup onion, chopped
- 1 small red bell pepper, diced
- ¼ teaspoon ground caraway
- 4 teaspoons red wine vinegar
- 2 tablespoons tomato paste
- Salt to taste
- Pepper to taste

Instructions:

1. Sprinkle salt and pepper over the pork and place in the slow cooker.
2. Scatter onion, garlic, pepper and thyme over the pork.
3. Add caraway, paprika, Worcestershire sauce, broth, vinegar and tomato paste into a bowl. Mix well and pour over the pork.
4. Cover the pot and cook on low for 7 to 8 hours or on High for 3 to 4 hours.

5. Remove the pork with a slotted spoon and place on your cutting board. When cool enough to handle, shred the pork with a pair of forks.
6. Add the pork back into the pot. Stir well. Heat if desired.
7. Add sour cream. Stir and serve.

Italian Pork Tenderloin

Makes: 8 servings

Carbs per serving: 3.1 grams

Ingredients:

- 4 tablespoons olive oil
- ¼ cup fresh sage
- ¼ cup oil packed sun-dried tomatoes
- 1 cup chicken broth
- ½ teaspoon salt or to taste
- ½ cup prosciutto, chopped
- ¼ cup fresh parsley, chopped
- ½ cup onion, chopped
- 3 pounds pork tenderloin, cut into ½ inch strips
- 1 cup heavy cream
- 1 teaspoon black pepper powder or to taste

Instructions:

1. Place a large skillet over medium high heat. Add oil. When the oil is heated, add prosciutto, herbs, onion and dried tomatoes.
2. Add pork strips and cook until brown. Flip sides and cook until brown. Transfer into the slow cooker.
3. Add broth, cream salt and pepper and mix well.
4. Cover the pot. Cook on Low for 2-3 hours or until pork is tender.
5. Serve hot.

Arianna Brooks

North African Lamb Shanks

Makes: 5 servings

Carbs per serving: 5 grams

Ingredients:

- 1 lamb shank (16-24 oz.)
- ½ teaspoon garlic, minced
- ½ tablespoon olive oil
- 1 small onion, minced
- 1 teaspoon ground cumin
- 1 teaspoon smoked paprika
- ¼ teaspoon ground allspice
- ½ cup broth
- 1 tablespoon harissa
- ½ sea salt
- ½ can diced tomatoes
- 1 tablespoon lemon juice
- Black pepper powder to taste
- Sea salt to taste
- A handful fresh mint to garnish
- Yogurt to garnish

Instructions:

1. Place a pan over medium heat. Add oil. When the oil is heated, add lamb shank and cook until brown on all the sides.
2. Remove lamb and place in the slow cooker.
3. Add onions into the onion and garlic and sauté until translucent. Stir in the cumin, paprika and allspice and sauté until aromatic.

4. Pour stock in the pan. Scrape the bottom of the pan to remove any brown bits that may be stuck to the pan.
5. Transfer into the slow cooker. Add tomatoes, lemon juice, harissa, salt and pepper and mix well.
6. Cover the pot and cook on Low for 6 to 7 hours or on High for 3-3 ½ hours or until meat is cooked.
7. Garnish with yogurt and parsley and serve.

Arianna Brooks

Moroccan Lamb Shoulders

Makes: 8 servings

Carbs per serving: 6.7 grams

Ingredients:

For Moroccan lamb shoulders

- 4 pounds lamb shoulder
- ½ pound carrot
- ½ cup fresh mint leaves, chopped
- 4 tablespoons Moroccan spice rub
- 1 medium onion, chopped
- ½ cup low sodium beef broth or water

For Moroccan spice rub

- ½ teaspoon ground ginger
- ½ teaspoon turmeric powder
- ½ teaspoon garlic powder
- ½ teaspoon cumin powder
- ½ teaspoon paprika
- ½ teaspoon red pepper flakes
- ¼ teaspoon coriander powder
- ¼ teaspoon ground cloves
- ¼ teaspoon black pepper powder
- ¼ teaspoon ground cinnamon
- ¼ teaspoon ground nutmeg
- ¼ teaspoon salt or to taste

Instructions:

1. To make Moroccan spice rub: Add all the ingredients of Moroccan spice rub into a bowl and stir. Add water or broth into the slow cooker. Rub the Moroccan spice rub all over the lamb and place in the slow cooker.
2. Place vegetables over the lamb and scatter mint leaves.
3. Cover the pot and cook on Low for 6-8 hours or on High for 3 to 4 hours.

Arianna Brooks

Lamb Curry

Makes: 3 servings

Carbs per serving: 11 grams (without rice)

Ingredients:

- ¾ pound lamb stew meat
- ½ inch ginger, minced
- 2 cloves garlic, minced
- ¼ cup coconut milk
- Salt to taste
- 7 oz. canned diced tomatoes
- Juice of a lime
- 1 ½ medium carrots, chopped
- A handful fresh cilantro, chopped
- 1 small zucchini, chopped
- 1 small onion, chopped
- ¾ teaspoon garam masala
- 2 tablespoons ground coriander
- ½ teaspoon turmeric powder
- 1 teaspoon chili powder
- 2 tablespoons ghee
- Black pepper to taste
- ½ cup water

Instructions:

1. Add garlic, ginger, salt, pepper, lime juice and coconut milk into a large bowl and mix well. Cover and refrigerate for 1-4 hours.
2. Place a skillet over medium heat. Add ghee. When ghee melts, add onions and sauté until golden brown.

Transfer into the slow cooker. Add meat and the chilled mixture.
3. Add rest of the ingredients and stir.
4. Cover the pot and cook on Low for 7 to 8 hours or on High for 3 ½ -4 hours.
5. Garnish with cilantro and serve with brown rice or cauliflower rice.

Arianna Brooks

Spanish Lamb with Sherry, Honey & Peppers

Makes: 3 servings

Carbs per serving: 12 grams (without serving options)

Ingredients:

- 1.1 pounds lamb shoulder, trimmed of excess fat, cut into cubes
- 1 medium onion, chopped
- ½ yellow bell pepper, sliced
- ½ red bell pepper, sliced
- ½ green bell pepper, sliced
- 1 tablespoon olive oil
- 1 clove garlic, grated
- 4.2 oz. medium sherry
- A pinch saffron strands
- 2 teaspoons honey
- 1 tablespoon chopped almonds, to garnish
- 1 tablespoon chopped parsley, to garnish
- 4.2 oz. lamb stock
- ½ tablespoon sherry vinegar
- Salt to taste
- Pepper to taste

Instructions:

1. Dry the lamb by patting with paper towels.
2. Place a skillet over medium heat. Add ½ tablespoon oil. When the oil is heated, add lamb and cook until brown all over. Remove with a slotted spoon and place in the slow cooker.
3. Add ½ tablespoon oil. When the oil is heated, add onion and sauté until light brown.

Slow Cooker Low Carb

4. Add bell peppers and cook for a couple of minutes. Add garlic and paprika and sauté for a few seconds until aromatic. Add sherry and stir. Turn off the heat.
5. Add stock, salt, pepper, vinegar, saffron and honey and stir. Pour over the meat.
6. Cover the pot and cook on low for 7 hours or on high for 3 ½ hours. Uncover and cook for the last 20-30 minutes of cooking.
7. Garnish with parsley and almonds and serve over any low carb option like cauliflower couscous or couscous if you have no issue with the carbs occasionally.

Arianna Brooks

Slow-Cooker Braised Pork with Salsa

Makes: 8 servings

Carbs per serving: 6 grams

Ingredients:

- 1 1/2 cups prepared tomatillo salsa (or you can use salsa verde)
- 3 pounds pork butt or shoulder (boneless)
- 1 finely sliced medium onion
- 3 finely sliced plum tomatoes (around 1/2 pound)
- 1 3/4 cups reduced-sodium chicken broth
- 1/2 cup reduced-fat sour cream
- 1/2 cup fresh cilantro (chopped), divided
- 1 teaspoon ground cumin
- Nonstick cooking spray

Instructions:

1. Trim the surface fat of the meat and discard it. Slice the meat apart following the fat layers around the muscles. Trim and discard the fat surfaces.
2. Chop them into 2-inch chunks and rinse thoroughly with cold water.
3. Grease the inside of the slow cooker with a cooking spray and place the pork chunks in it.
4. Set the heat to high and let it cook uncovered until you finish with the sauce.
5. Take a saucepan and combine the salsa, onion, chicken broth and ground cumin in it.
6. Bring the contents to boil over high heat and pour this hot mixture over the meat chunks.

7. Add the tomatoes and stir the contents gently until the flavors are incorporated.
8. Cover the cooker and cook for 7 hours until the meat is tender and soft
9. Once the cooking cycle is over, transfer the cooked meat to a large bowl and set aside
10. Take a large skillet and pour the cooking liquid (sauce + vegetables) from the slow cooker.
11. Bring the contents to boil over high heat and skim the fat from time to time. You will keep getting the froth as it boils, keep skimming.
12. After around 20 minutes, the sauce will begin to thicken and the flavors will also intensify.
13. Now, add the meat chunks and 1/4-cup cilantro to the pan and heat it through.
14. Transfer to a bowl and add a dollop of sour cream when you serve.
15. Sprinkle the remaining cilantro if you like and enjoy!

Arianna Brooks

Sage-Scented Pork Chops

Makes: 6 servings

Carbs per serving: 12 grams

Ingredients:

- 2 teaspoons crushed dried sage
- 10 boneless pork loin chops (about 3½ pounds), cut 3/4 inch-thick
- 1/2 medium head green cabbage (cut into 1/2-inch strips)
- 1/2 cup reduced-sodium chicken broth
- 1 finely sliced medium onion
- 1/3 cup apple juice
- 3 tablespoons crushed quick-cooking tapioca
- 2 tablespoons olive oil
- 1 teaspoon caraway seeds
- 1 teaspoon black pepper (ground)
- 1/2 teaspoon salt
- Fresh sage sprigs
- 1 tablespoon Dijon mustard
- Nonstick cooking spray

Instructions:

1. Trim the fat from the pork chops and set aside.
2. Take a small bowl and mix together the dried sage, black pepper and salt until well-combined
3. Rub this sage-pepper mixture to one side of the meat chunks and set aside.

4. Heat oil in an extra-large skillet over medium heat and add the one-side sage coated pork chunks to it (in batches).
5. Cook the meat until browned on both side and set aside.
6. Grease the inside of the slow cooker with nonstick cooking spray.
7. Place the onion in the bottom of the cooker and add the broth to it.
8. Add the apple juice, crushed tapioca and the browned chops to the cooker.
9. Top it with a layer of cabbage and cover the cooker.
10. Cook on high for 2.5 hours or on low heat for 5 hours.
11. Once the cooking cycle is over, transfer the meat chunks to a plate and cover it with aluminum foil. Set aside
12. Transfer the onions and cabbage from the cooker using a slotted spoon to a serving bowl.
13. Add the caraway seeds and mustards to the cooking liquid in the slow cooker.
14. Add pepper to the sauce if you desire and mix well.
15. Remove the foil from the plate and transfer some of the pork chops to the onion-cabbage mixture in the serving bowl.
16. Pour the sauce over it and garnish with fresh sage if you like.
17. Serve warm and enjoy!

Arianna Brooks

Mushroom-Sauced Pork Chops

Makes: 6 servings

Carbs per serving: 12 grams

Ingredients:

- 10.75 ounces condensed cream of mushroom soup (1 can), reduced-fat and reduced-sodium
- 4 pork loin chops (about 2 pounds), cut 3/4- inch thick
- 1 finely sliced small onion
- 1 1/2 cups fresh mushrooms (sliced)
- 3/4 teaspoon crushed dried thyme
- 2 tablespoons quick-cooking tapioca (crushed)
- 1 1/2 teaspoons Worcestershire sauce
- 1 tablespoon olive oil
- 1/2 cup apple juice or apple cider vinegar
- Fresh thyme sprigs
- 1/4 teaspoon garlic powder

Instructions:

1. Trim the fat from the pork chops and set aside.
2. Heat oil in a large skillet over medium heat and add the trimmed pork chops when the oil is hot.
3. Cook the meat until browned evenly on all the sides.
4. Drain the fat from the skillet and set aside
5. Place the onion in the bottom of the slow cooker and add the browned pork chops over it.
6. Take a medium bowl and combine the garlic powder, dried thyme, apple juice, Worcestershire sauce, crushed tapioca and mushroom cream soup. Mix them well until the flavors blend.

7. Add the chopped mushrooms to the sauce mixture and stir well until combined.
8. Pour this mixture over the pork chops in the slow cooker.
9. Cover the cooker and cook on high heat for 4.5 hours. If you are cooking on low heat, cook for 9 hours.
10. Transfer to a plate, garnish with thyme sprigs and serve warm.

Arianna Brooks

Slow-Cooker Baby Back Ribs

Makes: 6 servings

Carbs per serving: 13 grams

Ingredients:

- 3 pounds baby back pork ribs
- 3/4 cup ketchup
- 1 tablespoon apple cider vinegar
- 1 teaspoon onion powder
- 1 tablespoon brown sugar
- 1 teaspoon garlic powder
- 1 1/2 teaspoons smoked paprika
- 1/2 teaspoon crushed red pepper
- 1/2 teaspoon ground black pepper
- 1/4 teaspoon salt

Instructions:

1. Take a small bowl and combine the ketchup, apple cider vinegar, smoked paprika, crushed red pepper and brown sugar.
2. Whisk the contents together until they blend well and set aside
3. Take another small bowl and mix together onion powder, garlic powder, black pepper and salt.
4. Rup this garlic-pepper mixture over the meat and keep ready.
5. Take one tablespoon of the ketchup mixture and spread it over the brawny side of ribs.

Slow Cooker Low Carb

6. Place the coated ribs in the slow cooker and spread the remaining ketchup mixture over the other side of the ribs.
7. Cover the cooker and cook on high for 4 hours and on low heat for 8 hours.
8. Preheat the broiler to high and layer a baking tray with parchment paper.
9. Transfer the cooked meat to the baking tray and spoon the sauce mixture from the cooker and spread it over the meat.
10. Place this under the broiler and let it broil for 6 minutes until brown.
11. Carve the rack of the ribs between the bones and serve warm

Arianna Brooks

Slow-Cooker Char Siu Pork

Makes: 10 servings

Carbs per serving: 8 grams

Ingredients:

- 4 pounds trimmed boneless pork shoulder
- 4 scallions + extra for serving (cut into 1-inch pieces)
- 3 grated garlic cloves
- 2 tablespoons dry sherry or Shao Hsing rice wine
- 1 tablespoon dark sesame oil (toasted)
- 2 tablespoons dark soy sauce
- 1 tablespoon fresh ginger (grated)
- 2 tablespoons reduced-sodium soy sauce
- 2 tablespoons plum sauce
- 3/4 teaspoon five-spice powder (or all-spice powder)
- 2 tablespoons honey
- 1/2 cup water
- Sesame seeds, to garnish

Instructions:

1. Combine the scallions, rice wine, dark sesame oil, dark soy sauce, reduced-sodium soy sauce, grated ginger, plum sauce, honey, five-spice powder and water in a slow cooker.
2. Mix well until the flavors blend well. Add the trimmed pork and toss it over.
3. Use a spatula and turn the meat over the sauce couple of time to completely coat the meat with sauce.
4. Cover the cooker and cook on high for 4 hours and on low heat for 8 hours

5. Once the cooking cycle is over, remove the meat and place it on a cutting board.
6. Transfer the cooking liquid from the cooker carefully to a large measuring cup. Let it sit for 10 minutes
7. When the fat starts floating in the surface, skim it off from the liquid.
8. Heat a large skillet over high heat and pour the liquid through a fine sieve into the hot skillet.
9. Bring it to boil and continue for 15 minutes until the liquid gets the syrupy consistency
10. Shred the cooked meat on the cutting board using two forks and transfer to a plate.
11. Pour the syrupy sauce over the meat and serve with sesame seeds and scallions. Enjoy!

Arianna Brooks

Fennel & Pork Stew

Makes: 8 servings

Carbs per serving: 9 grams

Ingredients:

- 8 cups thinly sliced fennel (3 medium fennel bulbs should do) + 1/4 cup fronds (chopped)
- 2 1/2 pounds fat-trimmed pork shoulder (cut into 2-inch chunks)
- 3/4 cup Sauvignon Blanc dry white wine (or any similar variety white wine)
- 1 finely sliced medium onion
- 28 ounces drained whole tomatoes (1 can)
- 4 minced garlic cloves
- 1 tablespoon fresh rosemary (finely chopped)
- 1 1/2 teaspoons kosher salt, divided
- 2 teaspoons fresh oregano (finely chopped)
- 1 1/2 teaspoons black pepper (freshly ground), divided
- 2 tablespoons extra-virgin olive oil, divided

Instructions:

1. Layer the onion and fennel slices evenly in the slow cooker.
2. Cover the fennel fronds and refrigerate.
3. Season the pork with 3/4 teaspoon of pepper and salt (each) and set aside.
4. Heat 1-tablespoon oil over medium-high heat in a large skillet.
5. Add half the pork to the hot and oil and cook for 5 minutes until brown.

Slow Cooker Low Carb

6. Transfer the browned pork to the slow cooker and repeat step 5 with the remaining pork.
7. Transfer the remaining browned pork to the slow cooker.
8. Add wine to the skillet that you used to cook the pork and scrape the browned bits. Stir the wine and scraped bits. Turn off the heat.
9. Add the remaining black pepper and salt along with oregano, garlic and rosemary to the pork in the slow cooker.
10. Layer the drained tomatoes over the meat and pour the wine into the cooker from the skillet.
11. Cover the cooker and cook on high for 5 hours or on low heat for 8 hours.
12. Once the cooking cycle is over, open the cooker and stir the stew until well combined.
13. Transfer to a bowl and garnish with the refrigerated fennel fronds.
14. Serve hot and enjoy!

Arianna Brooks

Chinese Pork & Vegetable Hot Pot

Makes: 6 servings

Carbs per serving: 14 grams

Ingredients:

- 2 1/4 pounds trimmed boneless pork shoulder (cut into 1 1/2-inch chunks)
- 2 peeled medium white turnips (cut into ¾ inch-wide wedges
- 2 cups baby carrots
- 1 bunch scallions (separately sliced white and green parts)
- 2 tablespoons fresh ginger (minced)
- 14 ounces reduced-sodium chicken broth (1 can)
- 1/4 cup reduced-sodium soy sauce
- 4 minced garlic cloves
- 1 teaspoon aniseed
- 3 tablespoons medium sherry
- 2 teaspoons Chinese chili-garlic sauce
- 2 tablespoons toasted sesame seeds, for garnishing
- 1 tablespoon rice vinegar
- 4 teaspoons cornstarch + 2 tablespoons water (mix them together and set aside)
- 4 teaspoons brown sugar
- 1/2 cup water
- 1 cinnamon stick
- Nonstick cooking spray

Instructions:

1. Grease the insides of the slow cooker with a nonstick cooking spray.
2. Place the turnips and carrots in the bottom of the cooker.
3. Spread the pork and sliced scallion whites on top of the veggies
4. Head a saucepan over medium-high heat and pour the broth when the pan is hot.
5. Add water, medium sherry, vinegar, soy sauce, chili-garlic sauce, minced ginger, brown sugar and garlic to the saucepan.
6. Mix the contents well and bring it to boil. Pour this hot mixture over the veggies and meat.
7. Add the cinnamon stick and aniseed into the stew mixture. Cover the cooker.
8. Cook on high for 3.5 hours or on low heat for 6 hours until the meat and veggies become tender.
9. Once the cooking cycle is over, remove the cinnamon stick and aniseed from the cooker.
10. If you see any fat over the surface of the stew, skim it off and add the cornstarch mixture to the stew
11. Cover the cooker and cook on high for 15 minutes until the liquid thickens. You can stir once or twice in between.
12. Transfer to a bowl and sprinkle the sesame seeds and scallion greens over it.
13. Serve warm and enjoy!

Arianna Brooks

Hoisin Pork in Lettuce cups

Makes: 3 servings

Carbs per serving: 11 grams

Ingredients:

- 1 ¼ pounds boneless pork shoulder, trimmed of fat, cut into 2 inch pieces
- 2 tablespoon low sodium soy sauce
- ½ tablespoon packed dark brown sugar
- ½ tablespoon fresh ginger, grated
- 1 tablespoon chili garlic sauce
- 1 ½ tablespoon Hoisin sauce
- 1 small carrot, shredded
- 2 tablespoon fresh cilantro, chopped
- 2 scallions, white and green parts, finely chopped
- 1 dozen large lettuce cups.

Instructions:

1. Place the pork in the slow cooker along with soy sauce, brown sugar, ginger, and ½ tablespoon chili garlic sauce.
2. Cover and cook on low for 6 hours or until done.
3. In a large bowl, add ½ tablespoon chili garlic sauce, Hoisin sauce, carrot, cilantro, and scallions. Add pork to this along with a little of the remaining liquid in the pot. Mix well. If the mixture is too dry, then add some more of the liquid.
4. Shape the lettuce into cups and fill the pork mixture into it. Serve the lettuce cups.

Mushroom and Pork Chops

Makes: 3 servings

Carbs per serving: 8 grams

Ingredients:

- 5 oz. low sodium cream of mushroom soup
- 1/2 cup chopped onion
- 3 boneless pork loin chops
- 4 oz. sliced mushrooms
- 1/2 tsp Worcestershire sauce

Instructions:

1. Brown the pork loin chops in a greased skillet over medium high flame. Set aside.
2. Combine the mushrooms, onions, and soup in a bowl. Add the Worcestershire sauce and stir to mix. Ladle half of the mixture into the slow cooker.
3. Arrange the pork chops in the slow cooker, then arrange the pork chops inside. Pour the rest of the sauce on top of the pork chops.
4. Cover and cook for 4 hours on low or until the pork becomes very tender.

Arianna Brooks

Oriental Pork Roast

Makes: 4 servings

Carbs per serving: 4 grams

Ingredients:

- 1 1/2 lb. pork loin roast
- 1/4 cup low sodium soy sauce
- 1/4 cup sherry
- 1/4 tsp minced garlic
- 1/2 tsp ground ginger
- 1/2 tsp thyme
- 1/2 Tbsp. dry mustard

Instructions:

1. Put the pork roast inside a resalable plastic bag, then place this inside a deep bowl.
2. Combine the ginger, thyme, mustard, garlic, sherry, and soy sauce very well, then pour the mixture into the bag with the pork roast. Turn several times to coat, then refrigerate overnight or for 3 hours at least.
3. Put the pork roast and marinade inside the slow cooker, then cover and cook for 3 hours on high.
4. Take the roast out of the slow cooker and let it stand to cool down a bit. Chop it up and serve.

Slow Cooker Low Carb

Leg of Lamb

Makes: 3 servings

Carbs per serving: 1.8 grams

Ingredients:

- 2 ¼ pounds leg of lamb
- 3 cloves garlic, sliced
- 1 tablespoon olive oil + extra if needed
- 1 tablespoon fresh rosemary, remove stem and chopped or 1 tablespoon dried rosemary
- Salt to taste
- Pepper powder to taste
- 2 cups low sodium vegetable stock
- 6 tablespoon low sodium soy sauce

Instructions:

1. Make small cuts on leg of lamb. Stuff garlic slices in each of the cuts.
2. Apply olive oil and rosemary all over the lamb. Rub well. Sprinkle salt and pepper.
3. Place a large nonstick pan over medium heat. Add the leg of lamb. Cook until browned.
4. Meanwhile pour stock and soy sauce into the slow cooker. Add the browned lamb to the cooker.
5. Cover and cook on low for 8-10 hours.
6. When done, cool slightly. Slice and serve.

Arianna Brooks

Apple and Cranberry Pork Roast

Makes: 4 servings

Carbs per serving: 14 grams

Ingredients:

- 1/2 Tbsp. canola oil
- 1 1/2 lb. pork loin roast
- 1 1/2 cups sliced apples
- 1 cup apple juice
- 1/2 cup cranberries
- 1/8 tsp black pepper

Instructions:

1. Place a skillet over medium high flame and heat the canola oil. Brown the pork roast on all sides, then transfer into the slow cooker.
2. Add the rest of the ingredients into the slow cooker, then cover and cook for 6 hours on low.

Pork Chops in Beer

Makes: 3 servings

Carbs per serving: 7 grams

Ingredients:

- 1/2 Tbsp. olive oil
- 1 cup chopped onion
- 3 pork loin chops
- 6 oz. beer
- 1/2 tsp thyme

Instructions:

1. Place a large skillet over medium high flame and heat the olive oil. Cook the pork chops until browned on all sides. Set aside.
2. Arrange the onion inside the slow cooker, then place the pork chops on top.
3. In a bowl, mix together the thyme and beer, then pour this over the pork chops.
4. Cover and cook for 8 hours on low or for 4 hours on high.

Arianna Brooks

Lamb Stew

Makes: 3 servings

Carbs per serving: 10 grams

Ingredients:

- 1 lb. lean lamb, sliced into 1 inch cubes
- 1 Tbsp. olive oil
- 1/2 onion, sliced into wedges
- 1/4 tsp minced garlic
- 5 oz. low sodium cream of mushroom soup
- 1/4 cup water
- 1/4 tsp thyme
- 4 oz. fat free sour cream
- 1 Tbsp. flour

Instructions:

1. Place a skillet over medium high flame and heat the olive oil. Brown the lamb on all sides, then transfer into the slow cooker.
2. Using the same skillet, cook the onion and garlic until translucent and fragrant, then add the soup, thyme, and water and stir to combine. Scrape everything into the slow cooker.
3. Cover and cook for 8 hours on low, then increase heat to high. Combine the flour and cream and add 1/2 cup of the sauce from the slow cooker. Mix well, then pour it into the slow cooker and stir.
4. Cover and cook for 10 minutes, or until thick.

Lamb Paprikash

Makes: 3 servings

Carbs per serving: 10 grams

Ingredients:

- 1 lb. lamb, sliced into 1 inch pieces
- 7 oz. unsalted diced tomatoes
- 1/2 cup chopped onion
- 1/4 tsp minced garlic
- 1/2 tsp paprika
- 1/4 cup cold water
- 1/8 cup flour
- 1/4 cup fat free sour cream

Instructions:

1. Mix together the lamb, undrained tomatoes, garlic, paprika, and onion in the slow cooker.
2. Cover and cook for 8 hours on low, then increase the heat to high. Remove excess fat.
3. Combine the flour and cold water, then stir this into the mixture. Cover and cook for 20 minutes, or until thickened.
4. Take out about 1/4 cup of the liquid from the slow cooker and mix it with the sour cream in a bowl. Stir the mixture into the slow cooker and cook until heated.

Arianna Brooks

Maple Pork Ribs

Makes: 4 servings

Carbs per serving: 2.3 grams

Ingredients:

- ¼ tsp of ground allspice
- 2 lbs. of pork ribs (country-style)
- ¼ tsp of ground cinnamon
- ¼ cup of onion, diced
- 1 tbsp. of maple syrup (sugar-free)
- ½ tsp of garlic powder
- A dash of black pepper
- 1 tbsp. of soy sauce (low-sodium)
- ¼ tsp of ground ginger

Instructions:

1. In a mixing bowl, combine the allspice, cinnamon, onion, garlic powder, maple syrup, black pepper, ginger and soy sauce. Mix until properly combined then pour the mixture over the pork ribs inside the Crockpot.
2. Cook for 9 hours on low setting.

Slow Cooker Low Carb

Pork Stuffed Peppers

Makes: 6 servings

Carbs per serving: 14 grams

Ingredients:

- 6 medium green bell peppers
- 1 lb. of ground pork
- 2 cloves of garlic
- 1 medium onion, diced into small pieces
- 3 cups of cauliflower, chopped finely
- 6 oz. of tomato paste
- 1 cup of carrot, chopped finely
- 1 tbsp. of dried oregano flakes
- Kosher salt
- Black pepper
- 1 tsp of dried thyme
- 1 cup of chicken broth

Instructions:

1. Cut off the top part from the green bell peppers and remove the membranes and seeds. Place the peppers in the slow cooker with the open side facing up.
2. In a mixing bowl, combine the ground pork, onion, garlic, cauliflower, carrot, tomato paste, oregano flakes, salt, thyme and black pepper. Mix until all the ingredients are well incorporated.
3. Fill the bell peppers with the meat mixture then replace the tops. Once done, pour the chicken broth into the Crockpot.
4. Cover and cook for 8 hours on low setting.

Arianna Brooks

Tender and Tangy Pork Brisket

Makes: 10 servings

Carbs per serving: 14 grams

Ingredients:

- 4 lbs. of pork brisket, trimmed
- 1 cup of water
- 6 oz. of tomato puree
- 1 tbsp. of apple cider vinegar
- ½ tsp of dried thyme leaves, crushed
- 4 bay leaves
- 3 cloves of garlic, minced
- ½ tsp of black pepper
- 1 tsp of kosher salt

Instructions:

1. Place the pork brisket inside the slow cooker.
2. In a mixing bowl, combine the tomato puree, water, apple cider vinegar, bay leaves, dried thyme, kosher salt, garlic and black pepper.
3. Pour the mixture over the pork and make sure to coat the meat evenly.
4. Cover and cook for 8 hours on low setting.

Pork Adobado

Makes: 8 servings

Carbs per serving: 4.1 grams

Ingredients:

- ¼ cup of cilantro, for garnish
- Salt and pepper
- 2 bay leaves
- 1 tsp. of dried oregano
- 1 tsp. of cumin
- 1 tbsp. of coriander
- 1 onion, quartered
- 6 cloves of garlic
- 2 chipotles in adobo
- 3oz of New Mexico Chilies (dried)
- 3lbs of pork shoulder, fat trimmed

Instructions:

1. In a pan, add in the New Mexico chilies and cook for 5 minutes or until it is fragrant and starts to puff up as this brings out its full flavor. Once cool, remove the stems and seeds.
2. Prepare a small pot and fill it with water. Add in the New Mexico chilies and cover. Bring the liquid to a boil and let it simmer for about 5 minutes. Then, remove from the heat and don't remove from the pot for 30 minutes.
3. In a blender, add in the onion, oregano, garlic, coriander, cumin, chipotles, New Mexico chilies, and 1 cup of its cooking liquid. Process the ingredients together to make the adobo sauce.

4. Season the pork with the pepper and salt. Add in a small amount of the sauce into the slow cooker and place the pork on top. Then, pour the remaining adobo sauce on top of the meat.
5. Cover and cook for 8 hours. Using a fork, pull the meat apart and stir together with the adobo sauce. Serve on rice or on its own. Top with the cilantro before serving.

Pizza Meatloaf

Makes: 8 servings

Carbs per serving: 2 grams

Ingredients:

- Diced fresh parsley
- 1 cup of shredded mozzarella
- ½lb of hot pork sausage
- 1lb of ground beef
- ¼ tsp. of black pepper
- 1/3 cup of shaved parmesan
- ½ tbsp. of minced garlic
- ½ tsp. of Italian seasoning
- 1/3 cup of dry bread crumbs
- ½ cup of chopped green pepper
- ¼ cup of chopped onion
- 1 beaten egg
- 14oz of pizza sauce

Instructions:

1. Place 3 strips of foil into the slow cooker insert.
2. Take ½ cup of pizza sauce and set it aside. In a mixing bowl, combine the egg with the remaining pizza sauce. Then, stir in the black pepper, Parmesan, garlic, Italian seasoning, breadcrumbs, green pepper, and onion. Add in the pork sausage and ground beef and mix using hands.
3. Shape the mixture to make a loaf and place it inside the slow cooker on top of the aluminum foil strips. Cover and cook for 10 hours on low settings or 6 hours on high.

4. Once done, spread the reserved pizza sauce on the meat loaf and cover with mozzarella cheese. Cover and cook for another 15 minutes into the slow cooker. Then, remove the meat loaf using the foil strips and serve.

Lamb Chops

Makes: 8 servings

Carbs per serving: 5 grams

Ingredients:

- 1 large onion, sliced
- 2 teaspoons dried oregano
- 1 teaspoon dried thyme
- 1 teaspoon garlic powder
- ½ teaspoon salt or to taste
- ½ teaspoon pepper powder
- 16 lamb loin chops
- 6 cloves garlic, minced

Instructions:

1. Mix together oregano, thyme, garlic powder, salt and pepper. Rub this mixture over the lamb chops.
2. Place the onions in the slow cooker. Place the chops over the onions. Sprinkle garlic.
3. Cover and cook on low for 5-6 hours or until the meat is done.

Arianna Brooks

Pork Tenderloin

Makes: 3 servings

Carbs per serving: 1.7 grams

Ingredients:

- 1 ½ pounds lean pork tenderloin
- 1 cup nonfat chicken broth
- 2 garlic cloves, minced
- 1 teaspoon cumin
- ½ teaspoon paprika
- ½ teaspoon dried oregano
- 1 tablespoon Worcestershire sauce
- Salt to taste
- Pepper to taste

Instructions:

1. Add all the ingredients to the slow cooker.
2. Cover and cook on low for 7-8 hours or until done.
3. Slice and serve

Roasted Pork

Makes: 3 servings

Carbs per serving: 11 grams

Ingredients:

- 2 tablespoons low sodium soy sauce
- 2 tablespoons Hoisin sauce
- 2 tablespoons ketchup
- 1 ½ tablespoon honey
- 1 teaspoon garlic, minced
- 1 teaspoon fresh ginger, garlic
- ½ teaspoon dark sesame oil
- ½ teaspoon 5 spice powder
- 1 pound boneless pork shoulder, trimmed of fat
- ¼ cup fat free, low sodium chicken broth

Instructions:

1. Add all the ingredients except the broth and pork to a bowl. Whisk well. Pour this mixture into a large zip lock plastic bag.
2. Add pork to the bag. Seal and shake well. Place in the refrigerator for marinating for a minimum of 2 hours. Turn around the bag a couple of times.
3. Transfer the contents of the bag to the slow cooker.
4. Cover and cook on low for 8 hours. Remove pork with a slotted spoon from the cooker and place on a cutting board. Cover and keep it warm.
5. Add broth to the cooker. Cover and cook for 30 minutes or until the sauce is thick.

6. To serve, shred the pork with forks and pour sauce over it.

Simple Pork Chops

Makes: 2 servings

Carbs per serving: 4.3 grams

Ingredients:

- 2 pork loin chops
- 1/2 Tbsp. olive oil
- 1/2 cup sliced onion
- 1/2 cup low sodium chicken broth

Instructions:

1. Heat the olive oil in a large skillet over medium high flame. Cook the pork chops until browned on all sides.
2. Lightly grease the slow cooker and place the sliced onion inside.
3. Put the browned pork chops on top of the onions, then pour the chicken broth on top of.
4. Cover and cook for 5 hours on low, then serve.

Arianna Brooks

Camitas

Makes: 8 servings

Carbs per serving: 1.3 grams

Ingredients:

- 2 ½ lbs. pork shoulder, lean, fat trimmed
- 1 pc onion, diced
- 1 tsp oregano
- 3-4 clove garlic, minced
- 1 tsp cumin
- 1-2 chipotle peppers, diced
- 2 tbsp. of adobo sauce
- 3/4 cup of chicken broth or light beer
- 3/4 tsp salt
- 1/2 tsp. pepper
- 1-2 bay leaf

Instructions:

1. Season the meat with some salt & pepper.
2. Put the meat inside the crockpot.
3. Combine the rest of the ingredients in a medium-sized bowl and mix well. Pour the mixture all over the meat in the crockpot.
4. Allow to cook for about 6 to 8 hours on low heat setting or until the fork becomes tender enough to shred easily using a fork.
5. Pre-heat the oven at 500 degrees. Arrange the pork on one layer on top of a nonstick baking sheet. Let the meat roast for about 4 to 5 minutes, or just until the edges become toasted and crispy.

6. Slice the pork and serve immediately.

Arianna Brooks

Paprika Pork Tenderloin

Makes: 8 servings

Carbs per serving: 2.4 grams

Ingredients:

- 1 ½ lbs. pork tenderloin
- 1/2 cup of salsa of your choice
- 1 cup of chicken stock
- 1 tbsp. of oregano
- 2 tbsp. of smoked paprika
- 1/2 tsp salt
- Black pepper, to taste

Instructions:

1. Get a small-sized bowl and stir the chicken stock, paprika, oregano, salt & pepper, and salsa together.
2. Add the fat-trimmed meat to the slow cooker. Next pour the sauce over the meat and allow to cook for about 4 hours on high heat setting.
3. Using 2 forks shred the meat and cook without the lid on for we minutes more just to make sure that all the juices and flavors are absorbed.

Cochinita Pibil

Makes: 8 servings

Carbs per serving: 4.1 grams

Ingredients:

- 3 lbs of lean pork shoulder, fat trimmed
- 1/2 cup of orange juice
- 2 habaneros, seeded & diced
- 3 cloves garlic, diced
- 1 onion, cut into quarters
- 1 tsp of cumin
- 1 tsp of dried oregano
- 1 tbsp. of coriander
- 4 tbsp. of Achiote paste
- 1/2 cup of chicken broth
- 1/2 cup of apple cider vinegar
- Salt & pepper
- 1/4 cup of cilantro, for garnishing

Instructions:

1. Season the meat with some salt & pepper. Afterwards, rub Achiote paste on the outside of the meat.
2. Spread out the garlic and onions at the slow cooker's bottom, as evenly as possible, and then put the meat on top.
3. Get a small bowl and mix all the remaining unused ingredients. Mix well and then pour on top of the pork shoulder.

4. Allow 6 to 8 hours for slow cooking or until the fork is tender enough to shred easily. Using a fork, pull the meat apart and combine it with the sauce.
5. Serve the dish as is, or with rice. You can also serve it as a sandwich (spicy pulled pork sandwich) or in a taco. Garnish the pork with fresh chopped cilantro.

Lamb Shanks w/ Cannellini Beans

Makes: 12 servings

Carbs per serving: 12.9 grams

Ingredients:

- 4 pcs. Lamb shanks (1 ½ lb. each)
- 1 (19 oz.) can cannellini or any other type of white beans, rinsed & drained
- 1 cup onions, chopped
- 1 1/2 cups carrots, diced & peeled
- 3/4 cup celery, chopped
- 2 cloves garlic, sliced thinly
- 3 tsp dried tarragon
- 1/2 tsp salt
- 1/4 tsp black pepper, freshly ground
- 2 (28 oz.) can of tomatoes, diced and undrained

Instructions:

First, make sure to trim the fat off the lamb shanks.

1. Put the beans, carrots, onions, garlic, and celery in a 7-qt slow cooker. Mix the ingredients well.
2. Put the lamb shanks on top of the bean mixture, sprinkled with tarragon, and salt & pepper. Then, pour the tomatoes on top of the shanks.
3. Put the cooker lid on and allow to cook for 1 hour on high heat setting.
4. After an hour, adjust the heat to low setting, and cook for 9 hours more or just until the shanks become tenderized.
5. Take the lamb shanks out of the slow cooker.

6. Pour the bean mixture in the cooker through a sieve or colander to collect the liquid. Set the liquid aside and let it stand of around 5 minutes before skimming the fat off its surface.
7. Combine the bean mixture with the skimmed liquid.
8. Remove the bones from the lamb shanks. Discard the bones.
9. Serve the lamb dish with the bean mixture.
10. Enjoy while hot.

Note:

If you are unable to prepare the dried beans, canned beans is a convenient option, but the sodium content may be a drawback. However, you can lower the sodium content of any type of commercially-available canned beans by as much as 40% just by carefully draining and then properly rinsing them.

Amazing Slow Cooked Pork Tenderloin

Makes: 10 servings

Carbs per serving: 2.3 grams

Ingredients:

- 2 lb. pork tenderloin
- 1 cup of water
- 1 pack of onion soup mix, dry
- 1/2 cup of white wine
- 3 tbsp. of low sodium soy sauce
- 3 tbsp. of garlic, minced
- Pepper, to taste

Instructions:

1. Put the pork tenderloin inside the slow cooker together with the onion soup pack contents. Pour the wine, soy sauce, and water on top of the meat. Turn the meat around to coat on all sides.
2. Spread the garlic carefully on the pork. Leave as much garlic as possible at the top of the meat while cooking. Sprinkle some pepper.
3. Put the cooker lid in place. Cook for about 4 hours on low heat setting.
4. Serve with the cooking liquid on the side as dipping or au jus.
5. Enjoy while warm.

Arianna Brooks

Pork with Beans & Greens

Makes: 8 servings

Carbs per serving: 11.7 grams

Ingredients:

For the Spice Rub

- 1 tbsp. chili powder
- 1/2 tsp red pepper, flaked
- 1/2 tsp sea salt or kosher

For the Dish

- 2 lbs. pork shoulder, w/ all visible fat trimmed
- 3 cloves of garlic, halved
- 1 cup of chicken stock, low sodium
- 2 (14.5 oz.) cans of cannellini beans, drained & rinsed
- 1 (14.5 oz.) can of low-sodium diced tomatoes
- 2 cups kale or escarole, chopped
- 1/2 cup of pepitas (shelled pumpkin seeds that can be found in supermarkets along the nuts aisle.

Instructions:

1. Make the spice rub by mixing the red pepper, salt, and chili powder together.
2. Rub the mixture all over the pork the night before or at least an hour before the intended cooking time.
3. Refrigerate until it is time to cook.
4. Put the pork inside the slow cooker together with the garlic.

5. Pour the chicken stock on the pork, then allow to cook for about 5 to 6 hours over low heat setting.
6. Take the cooker lid off, and break the meat up into big chunks.
7. Put the tomatoes, kale, and beans in the cooker. Allow 1 more hour to cook.
8. Get a dry skillet and toast the pepitas.
9. Topped with pepitas, serve the dish immediately as it is best consumed warm.

Arianna Brooks

Diet Cola Pot Roast

Makes: 12 servings

Carbs per serving: 5.4 grams

Ingredients:

- 3 lbs. pot roast
- 2 cans of 10 3/4 oz. low sodium, fat-free cream of mushroom soup
- 1 pack of onion soup mix, dry
- 2 cans 16 oz. diet cola (or diet ginger ale, depending on preference)

Instructions:

1. Put the meat inside the slow cooker.
2. Get a large-sized bowl and combine the cola, soup mix, and dry mix.
3. Pour over the meat in the slow cooker and allow to cook for about 6 hours over high heat. If desired, you can add more potatoes and carrots 2 to 3 hours before the end of set cooking time.
4. Remove from the cooker.
5. Best served with egg noodles or rice.

Slow Cooker Low Carb

Barbecue Pulled Pot Roast

Makes: 12 servings

Carbs per serving: 12.3 grams

Ingredients:

- 3 lbs. pork roast, boneless
- 1 cup celery, chopped
- 1 cup onions, chopped
- 1 cup of ketchup
- 1 cup of barbecue sauce
- 1 cup of water
- 2 tbsp. of vinegar
- 2 tbsp. of Worcestershire sauce
- 2 tbsp. of brown sugar
- 1 tsp chili powder
- 1 tsp salt
- 1/2 tsp pepper
- 1/2 tsp garlic powder

Instructions:

1. Put all the ingredients in the slow cooker, except for the pork roast.
2. Place the pork on top of the other ingredients.
3. Put the cooker cover in place. Cook for 6 to 7 hours on high heat setting.
4. Take the roast from the cooker, leaving the sauce behind. Shred the meat.
5. Put the shredded meat back into the cooker. If preferred, you can thicken the sauce a bit by simmering for a few minutes on the stovetop.
6. Best served with rice. Enjoy while hot.

Arianna Brooks

Cuban-Style Pot Roast

Makes: 10 servings

Carbs per serving: 2 grams

Ingredients:

- 3 lb. chuck roast, boneless
- 1/2 cup of salsa verde
- 1/2 cup of canned green chili, chopped
- 1 cup tomatoes, diced
- 2 tbsp. of dried onions, flaked
- 1 tsp of garlic powder
- 1/2 cup yellow and red peppers, sliced into thin strips
- 1 tsp salt
- 2 tbsp. of ground cumin
- 1 tbsp. of ground coriander
- 1 tsp of dried oregano
- 1 tbsp. of chili powder
- 1/2 tsp of black pepper
- 2 tbsp. of apple cider vinegar

Instructions:

1. Season the roast with a generous amount of salt & pepper.
2. In a hot pan, sear the pork roast until all sides are browned.
3. Put the roast at the bottom of a 5-qt crockpot.
4. Put the chili, salsa verde, and tomatoes in the same pan where the pork meat was seared.
5. Bring to a boil after deglazing. Pour the contents of the pan into the slow cooker, on top of the meat.

6. Add the garlic, onion flakes, cumin, salt & pepper, oregano, coriander, black pepper, apple cider vinegar, and chili powder in, and then stir well.
7. Allow to cook for about 4 hours on high heat setting, or about 6 hours on low to make sure that the meat is properly tenderized.
8. Remove the meat from the crockpot, shred, and immediately served with your preferred toppings.

Balsamic Bacon Meatloaf Barbecue

Makes: 10 servings

Carbs per serving: 7 grams

Ingredients:

- 1/2 cup of balsamic vinegar
- 1/4 cup of water
- 1 cup of ketchup (no sugar added)
- 1 tbsp. Worcestershire sauce (organic preferred)
- 1 tsp of maple extract
- 1/4 tsp of cumin
- 1/4 tsp of salt
- 1/2 tsp of pepper
- 1 tbsp. of cocoa powder, unsweetened
- 1/4 tsp of stevia extract, pure
- 2 1/2 lbs. turkey, ground
- 1 egg, beaten
- 1/2 cup of parmesan cheese
- 1 tsp cumin
- 1 tsp salt
- 1 tsp of garlic powder
- 1 tsp of smoked paprika
- 8 oz. bacon (sugar free)

Instructions:

1. Get a small bowl and then combine the first 5 ingredients on the list. Set the mixture aside.
2. Put in the next 5 ingredients on the list. Stir to blend with the ingredients that are already in the bowl.
3. Measure ½ cup of the resulting sauce mixture and spread it at the bottom of the slow cooker.

4. Get another large-sized bowl and mix together the egg, turkey, cheese, and dry seasonings until they are blended well. Set the mixture aside.
5. Put 5 or strips bacons in the crockpot, laid down side by side.
6. Put the ground turkey mixture on top of the bacon, creating a 10" oblong shape in the process.
7. Get the bottom parts of the bacon and fold on the side of the meatloaf. Top the meatloaf with the remaining pieces of bacon.
8. Pour the remaining sauce over the dish.
9. Put the crockpot cover in place, then allow to cook for about 8 hours on low setting or 4 hours on high.

Chapter Six - Main Course - Chicken and Turkey

Slow Cooked Tahini Chicken Thighs

Makes: 4 servings

Carbs per serving: 2 grams

Ingredients:

- 4 chicken thighs, skinless, boneless
- 1 ½ tablespoons extra virgin olive oil, divided
- 1 teaspoon lemon zest, grated
- 1 clove garlic, minced
- ¼ teaspoon salt
- 2 tablespoons tahini
- 3 teaspoons water
- 1 tablespoon lemon juice
- 1 small shallot, grated

Instructions:

1. Add ½ tablespoon oil into the slow cooker and spread it on the bottom of the pot.
2. Place chicken in it. Season with salt and pepper.
3. Add 1-tablespoon oil, lemon zest, garlic, salt, tahini, water, lemon juice and shallot into a bowl and whisk well.
4. Spoon this mixture over the chicken.
5. Cover the pot and cook on low for 6 hours or on high for 3 hours.
6. Garnish with parsley and serve.

Cherry Tomato Chicken Cacciatore

Makes: 2-3 servings

Carbs per serving: 2.8 grams (1 ½ pieces)

Ingredients:

- 1 ½ pounds bone-in chicken legs and thighs
- ½ teaspoon olive oil
- ½ pound cherry tomatoes
- Red pepper flakes to taste
- ½ teaspoon dried oregano
- ½ cup water
- ¼ cup green olives, pitted, rinsed, to garnish
- 1 clove garlic, crushed
- ½ -1 teaspoon salt
- 2 tablespoons tart red table wine
- A sprig fresh basil, torn, to garnish

Instructions:

1. Place the tomatoes in a ziplock bag. Leave a small hole and seal rest of the bag. Crush the tomatoes lightly with a meat mallet.
2. Place a skillet over medium heat. Add oil. When the oil is heated, add chicken and cook until brown. Transfer into the slow cooker.
3. Add rest of the ingredients and mix well.
4. Cover the pot and cook on low for 6 to 7 hours or on high for 3- 3 ½ hours.
5. Garnish with olives and basil and serve.

Chicken Lo Mein

Makes: 3 servings

Carbs per serving: 3.1 grams

Ingredients:

- ¾ pound chicken, skinless, boneless, sliced
- ½ bunch Bok Choy or Napa cabbage, sliced
- ½ teaspoon fresh ginger, minced
- 6 oz. Konaberry kelp noodles or kelp noodles
- 1 clove garlic, minced
- Black pepper powder to taste
- Salt to taste
- Cooking spray

For marinade

- ½ tablespoon coconut aminos or tamari
- ¼ teaspoon garlic, minced
- ¼ teaspoon sesame oil

For sauce

- 6 tablespoons chicken broth
- ½ tablespoon sukrin gold fiber syrup or any other sweetener of your choice
- ½ tablespoon rice vinegar
- ¼ teaspoon xanthan gum (optional)
- 1 teaspoon sesame oil
- 2 tablespoons coconut aminos or tamari
- ½ teaspoon red pepper flakes

Instructions:

1. Add all the ingredients of marinade into a bowl and stir. Add chicken into it and toss until chicken is well coated. Refrigerate for 30-60 minutes.
2. Grease the inside of the slow cooker by spraying with cooking spray.
3. Add chicken along with marinade.
4. Cover the pot and cook on low for 1 ½ -2 hours or on high for 45-60 minutes. Stir 1-2 times while it is cooking.
5. Remove the chicken from the cooker and set aside on a plate.
6. Add garlic, ginger and cabbage into the slow cooker and stir. Place chicken over it.
7. Mix together all the ingredients of the sauce in a bowl and pour into the slow cooker.
8. Cover the pot and cook on low for 1 hour or on high for 30 minutes. Stir 1-2 times while it is cooking.
9. Rinse kelp noodles during the last 10 minutes of cooking time. Soak it in water for 10 minutes. Drain.
10. Add noodles into the cooker. Add xanthan gum and carefully cover the noodles with the sauce with a pair of tongs.
11. Cook on High for 10-12 minutes.
12. Serve hot or warm in bowls.

Creamy Sundried Tomato Chicken

Makes: 4 servings

Carbs per serving: 10.8 grams

Ingredients:

- 2 tablespoons unmodified potato starch or cornstarch or tapioca starch
- Freshly ground black pepper to taste
- 1 ½ tablespoons extra virgin olive oil, divided
- 6 tablespoons sundried tomatoes (not packed in oil), sliced
- ½ teaspoon Italian seasoning
- ½ can coconut milk
- Few leaves fresh basil, shredded, to garnish
- Salt to taste
- 4 chicken thighs, bone-in, skinless
- 1 medium onion, thinly sliced
- ½ tablespoon garlic, minced
- Red pepper flakes to taste
- ½ cup chicken stock or broth

Instructions:

1. Add potato starch, salt and pepper into a shallow bowl. Dredge chicken in it.
2. Place a nonstick pan over medium heat. Add 1-tablespoon oil. When the oil is heated, add chicken and cook until brown on all the sides.
3. Remove chicken with a slotted spoon and place in the slow cooker.
4. Add ½ tablespoon oil into the pan. When the oil is heated, add onion and sauté until translucent.

5. Add sundried tomatoes, Italian seasoning, garlic and red pepper flakes and sauté for a few seconds until fragrant. Turn off the heat.
6. Add coconut milk and broth and stir. Pour over the chicken and stir.
7. Cover the pot and cook on low for 5-6 hours or on high for 2 ½ -3 hours.
8. Garnish with basil and serve.

Slow Cooker Chicken Creole

Makes: 8 servings

Carbs per serving: 13.8 grams

Ingredients:

- 8 chicken breast halves, skinless, boneless
- Creole seasoning blend to taste
- 2 stalks celery, diced
- 6 cloves garlic, minced
- 2 cans (4 ounces each) mushrooms, drained
- Salt to taste
- Pepper to taste
- 2 cans (14.5 ounces each) stewed tomatoes with its liquid
- 2 green bell peppers, chopped
- 2 onions, chopped
- 2 fresh jalapeño peppers, deseeded, chopped

For creole seasoning blend

- 3 tablespoons onion powder
- 3 tablespoons dried oregano
- 1 ½ tablespoons dried thyme
- 1 ½ tablespoons white pepper powder
- 7 ½ tablespoons paprika
- 3 tablespoons garlic powder
- 3 tablespoons dried basil
- 1 ½ tablespoons black pepper powder
- 1 ½ tablespoons cayenne pepper
- 4 ½ tablespoons salt

Instructions:

1. To make creole seasoning: Add onion powder, oregano, thyme, white pepper powder, paprika, garlic powder, basil, black pepper powder, salt and cayenne pepper into an airtight container. Stir and use as much as required in the recipe.
2. Seal the container with remaining seasoning and use the seasoning in some other recipe.
3. Lay the chicken in the slow cooker. Sprinkle salt, pepper and creole seasoning all over the chicken.
4. Add tomatoes, bell pepper, onion, jalapeño pepper, celery, garlic and mushrooms and mix until well combined.
5. Cover the pot and cook on low for 10-12 hours or on high for 5-6 hours.

Slow Cooker Jerk Chicken

Makes: 5 servings

Carbs per serving: 6 grams

Ingredients:

- 2 pounds skinless chicken legs (approximately 10 drumsticks)
- 1 cup green onions (chopped)
- 1 garlic clove
- 3/4 teaspoon thyme (dried)
- 1/4 teaspoon cayenne pepper
- 1/4 teaspoon ground cinnamon
- 1 teaspoon ground allspice seasoning blend
- 1 tablespoon honey
- 1 teaspoon dried mustard (ground)
- 1 teaspoon coconut oil or olive oil (for greasing)
- 1/2 teaspoon salt
- 1 tablespoon fresh Lemon Juice

Instructions:

1. Start by preparing the jerk seasoning
2. Add the chopped onions, garlic, dried thyme, cayenne pepper, cinnamon, allspice blend, honey, mustard and salt to a food processor
3. Pulse them together until the contents are thoroughly combined
4. Transfer to a bowl and set aside
5. Grease the slow cooker with coconut oil and place the chicken drumsticks in the bottom
6. Top the chicken pieces with the prepared jerk seasoning mixture

7. Use a spatula or large spoon to stir the chicken pieces well over the seasoning so that they are completely coated
8. Cook on low for 4 hours
9. Add the lemon juice over the chicken pieces as you turn them over after 2 hours (in between)
10. Once the cooking cycle is over, turn off the heat.
11. Set the oven to broil
12. Line a baking tray with parchment sheet and place the cooked chicken over it.
13. Pour out the juices that remain in the slow cooker over the chicken (add a splash of water to scrape the juices from the side and bottom)
14. Place the baking sheet in the oven and broil the chicken for 5 minutes until it turns crispy on the outside
15. Transfer to a serving plate and serve warm.

Slow Cooker Low Carb

Slow Cooker Chicken Fajitas

Makes: 6 servings

Carbs per serving: 7.5 grams

Ingredients:

- 2 pounds chicken breast halves (boneless and skinless)
- 1 halved and sliced large yellow onion
- 14.5 ounces petite diced tomatoes with green chilies (1 can)
- 4 minced garlic cloves
- 1 teaspoon paprika
- 1 julienned bell pepper (red, orange and green – 1 each)
- 3/4 teaspoon ground coriander
- 2 1/2 teaspoon chili powder
- 2 tablespoons fresh lime juice
- 2 teaspoons ground cumin
- 1 tablespoon honey
- 1 teaspoon salt
- 3/4 teaspoon pepper
- Nonstick cooking spray

For serving:

- Flour tortillas
- Sour cream (1 gallop)
- Cilantro (chopped)
- Cheddar cheese (shredded)

Arianna Brooks

Instructions:

1. Lightly grease the inside of the slow cooker
2. Transfer half of the canned tomatoes to the slow cooker and layer them in the bottom evenly
3. Top it with half of the chopped bell peppers, followed by half of the chopped onions.
4. Sprinkle the minced garlic over the top and top it with the chicken breasts
5. Take a medium-sized bowl and combine the paprika, chili powder, coriander, cumin, pepper and salt. Mix them well until blended
6. Sprinkle half of this seasoning evenly over the chicken breasts until the part is covered with it.
7. Flip the chicken breast and sprinkle the remaining seasoning over it evenly.
8. Now top it with the remaining half of the tomatoes followed by the bell peppers and finally the onions.
9. Cook on high for 4 hours or on low heat for 8 hours until the vegetables are tender and chicken is completely cooked through
10. Once the cooking cycle in the cooker is over, remove the chicken and shred it or cut into strips Set aside
11. Take out one cup of the broth from the slow cooker which is mostly the tomato liquid and discard the remaining liquid
12. Take a small bowl and add the honey and lime juice in it. Whisk them together until the flavors blend.
13. Place the chicken pieces back to the slow cooker and add this honey-lime juice mixture. Check for taste and add more salt or pepper if desired
14. Toss it gently and transfer to a plate.
15. Serve warm with tortillas and sour cream. Sprinkle some cilantro and shredded cheese for juicy taste.

16. Enjoy!

Arianna Brooks

Slow Cooker Balsamic Chicken

Makes: 4 servings

Carbs per serving: 13.8 grams

Ingredients:

- 8-10 chicken thighs (boneless, skinless)
- 8 ounces quartered white button mushrooms
- 16 ounces white pearl onions (frozen) – 1 package
- 3 tablespoons tomato paste
- 5 minced garlic cloves
- 3/4 cup balsamic vinegar
- 2 stems fresh rosemary
- 1 cup chicken stock
- 2 tablespoons extra-virgin olive oil
- 1/2 cup pomegranate seeds
- 1 bay leaf
- 1/4 cup brown sugar
- 1 tablespoon butter
- 1/4 cup torn or chopped parsley leaves (flat leaf)
- Kosher salt and freshly ground black pepper, to taste
- Nonstick cooking spray

Instructions:

1. Season the chicken thighs with black pepper and salt. Set them aside
2. Heat olive oil over medium-high heat in a large skillet and add the chicken thighs to it in batches
3. Stir-fry or sauté for 5 minutes until it turns golden brown. Flip the sides and sauté for 5 more minutes until browned.

Slow Cooker Low Carb

4. Repeat with the remaining batches of the chicken thighs, remove from heat and set aside
5. Grease the inside of the slow cooker with a nonstick cooking spray
6. Spread the pearl onions in the bottom of the cooker in even layer followed by the button mushrooms.
7. Top it with garlic, bay leaf and fresh rosemary stems.
8. Place the sautéed chicken over the top and set aside
9. Take a medium-sized bowl and combine the chicken stock, brown sugar, balsamic vinegar and tomato paste. Mix them well until combined. Add a bit of salt and pepper. Stir again.
10. Pour this stock-vinegar mixture over the chicken in the slow cooker
11. Cook on high for 3 hours, checking if the chicken is cooked in between after 1.5 hours.
12. Cook for 30 more minutes after the cooking cycle (3 hours) is done to ensure the chicken doesn't show any pink color.
13. Transfer the cooked chicken to a dish and cover it with an aluminum foil.
14. Take out the cooked vegetables from the slow cooker leaving behind the liquid. Remove the foil and add the vegetables to the chicken.
15. Take a saucepan and pour the liquid from the cooker into the pan. Let it cook for 5 minutes over medium heat until it comes to a low boil.
16. Wait until the liquid is reduced by half and add the butter to it. Reduce the heat and carefully whisk together the liquid and butter until the butter melts.
17. Once the sauce thickens, remove from heat and pour it over the chicken-veggie mixture.

18. Transfer to a plate and garnish with pomegranate seeds and parsley.
19. Serve warm with brown rice. Enjoy!

Buffalo Chicken Salads

Makes: 6 servings

Carbs per serving: 11 grams

Ingredients:

- 1/2 cup reduced-sodium Buffalo sauce or Buffalo chicken sauce
- 1 1/2 pounds chicken breast halves (skinless and boneless)
- 1 teaspoon Worcestershire sauce
- 2 chopped romaine hearts (center leaves of the romaine lettuce)
- 2 tablespoons blue cheese (crumbled)
- 1/3 cup light mayonnaise
- 1 cup croutons (whole grain)
- 1/2 cup red onion (finely sliced)
- 4 teaspoons apple cider vinegar
- 2 tablespoons milk (fat-free)
- 1 teaspoon paprika
- Nonstick cooking spray

Instructions:

1. Grease the slow cooker with a nonstick cooking spray
2. Layer the chicken in the bottom of the slow cooker and set aside
3. Take a small bowl and add the buffalo sauce, Worcestershire sauce and 2 teaspoons apple cider vinegar. Mix them together until they are thoroughly combined.

4. Pour this sauce-vinegar mixture over the chicken and sprinkle the paprika over the top.
5. Cover the cooker and cook on low for 4 hours.
6. Before the serving time, take a small bowl and place the light mayonnaise in it.
7. Add the fat-free milk and the remaining 2 teaspoons of apple cider vinegar. Whisk them together until well-combined
8. Add the blue cheese to this mixture and stir well until the flavors blend
9. Once the cooking cycle is over, pull out the cooked meat into easy-to-bite pieces using 2 forks
10. Take 6 plates and divide the romaine hearts among the plates. Transfer the chicken pieces to the leaves and pour a spoon of the sauce over it.
11. If you have blue cheese remaining, drizzle them over it and top it with red onion slices and croutons.
12. Serve immediately and enjoy.

Slow Cooker Low Carb

Rosemary Chicken

Makes: 6 servings

Carbs per serving: 8 grams

Ingredients:

- 1 1/2 pounds chicken thighs or breast halves (skinless and boneless)
- 2 teaspoons crushed dried rosemary
- 1/2 cup reduced-sodium chicken broth
- 9 ounces artichoke hearts (frozen), 1 package
- 1/2 cup onion (chopped)
- 12 minced garlic cloves
- 1 tablespoon cornstarch
- 1 teaspoon lemon zest (finely grated)
- 1 tablespoon cold water
- 1/2 teaspoon black pepper (ground)
- Lemon wedges (for garnishing)
- Nonstick cooking spray

Instructions:

1. Grease the inside of the slow cooker with a nonstick cooking spray and set aside.
2. Coat a large skillet with cooking spray and heat over medium heat.
3. Add half of the chicken into the hot skillet and brown on both sides. Similarly, add the remaining half of the chicken and brown. Turn off heat and set aside.
4. Place the frozen artichoke hearts in the slow cooker. Add the chopped onions and garlic cloves to it. Mix the contents until combined.

5. Take a small bowl and combine the rosemary, broth, pepper and lemon zest.
6. Pour this mixture over the vegetable mixture in the slow cooker.
7. Add the browned chicken into the cooker and using a spoon, take some of the liquid mixture lying in the cooker and pour it over the chicken.
8. Cover the cooker and cook on high for 3.5 hours or on low heat for 7 hours.
9. Once the cooking cycle is over, transfer the artichoke and chicken mixture to a plate. Reserve the cooking liquid.
10. Cover the plate with aluminum foil.
11. Take a small bowl and mix the cold water and cornstarch in it. Stir well until combined.
12. Pour this cornstarch mixture into the liquid in the cooker. Cover and cook on high for 15 minutes until the liquid thickens.
13. Pour a spoon of this sauce over the artichoke-chicken when you serve.
14. Add the lemon wedges and relish!

Slow Cooker Low Carb

Slow-Cooker Vietnamese Pulled Chicken

Makes: 12 servings

Carbs per serving: 8 grams

Ingredients:

- 3 cups low-sodium chicken broth
- 4 pounds chicken breasts (skin-on and bone-in)
- 3 finely sliced shallots,
- 2 cups carrots (grated or julienned)
- 4 finely sliced Thai chilies
- 1/4 cup fish sauce
- 1/3 cup fresh mint (sliced)
- 2 tablespoons brown sugar (lightly packed)
- 1 teaspoon red pepper (crushed)
- 1/3 cup fresh basil (sliced)
- 2 teaspoons lime zest
- 1/2 cup lime juice

Instructions:

1. Pour the chicken broth into the slow cooker and add shallots, chilies, fish sauce, brown sugar and lime zest to it. Stir once until combined.
2. Place the chicken in the cooker with its meat-side facing down in the broth.
3. Cover and cook on high for 3 hours and on low heat for 6 hours
4. Once the cooking cycle is over, remove the chicken from the cooker and place it on a clean cutting board.
5. Remove the skin and shred the meat using a fork or sharp knife.

6. Transfer the shredded chicken back to the slow cooker and add the carrots, mint, pepper and basil. Stir well until combined.
7. You can skip the step of adding pepper if you don't want your dish to be too hot.
8. Cover and cook on high for 15 minutes until the flavors blend well.
9. Transfer to a plate and serve warm. Enjoy!

Savory Barbecue Chicken

Makes: 4 servings

Carbs per serving: 15 grams

Ingredients:

- 10 skinned chicken drumsticks and/or thighs (around 2 to 2.5 pounds)
- 2 tablespoons jalapeño pepper jelly
- 2 tablespoons quick-cooking tapioca
- 4 slices bread (whole grain)
- 1/2 cup tomato sauce
- 1/4 teaspoon red pepper (crushed)
- 2 tablespoons lemon juice
- 1 teaspoon brown sugar
- 1 teaspoon cumin (ground)

Instructions:

1. Add the jalapeno pepper jelly, tapioca, tomato sauce, lemon juice, cumin, brown sugar and red pepper into the slow cooker.
2. Mix the contents thoroughly until well combined.
3. Place the chicken pieces on this sauce mixture with its meat-side facing down.
4. Cover the cooker and cook on high for 3.5 hours. If you are cooking on low, cook for 7 hours
5. Before you serve, toast the bread slices and transfer to a plate.
6. Once the cooking cycle is over, transfer the barbeque chicken to a bowl.

Arianna Brooks

Shredded Chicken Master Recipe

Makes: 12 servings

Carbs per serving: 0 grams

Ingredients:

- 5 pounds skinned chicken thighs
- 1/2 teaspoon black peppercorns (whole)
- 4 fresh thyme sprigs
- 32 ounces reduced-sodium chicken broth (1 carton)
- 4 fresh parsley stems
- 2 garlic cloves (sliced into half)
- 2 bay leaves
- Nonstick cooking spray
- Black pepper powder, for garnishing

Instructions:

1. Grease the inside of the slow cooker with a nonstick cooking spray and place the chicken thighs in the bottom. Set aside
2. Prepare the bouquet garni by placing the peppercorns, thyme sprigs, parsley stems, garlic and bay leaves in the center of a cheese cloth (should be double thick 8-inch square and 100 percent cotton)
3. Gather the corners of the cloth and close it together. Tie it with a kitchen string (100 percent cotton) tightly.
4. Place the bouquet garni in the slow cooker and pour the chicken broth all over the chicken and garni.
5. Cover the cooker and cook on high for hours. If you are cooking on low, set it for 8 hours.

6. Once the cooking cycle is over, remove the bouquet garni and discard it.
7. Transfer the cooked chicken to a large bowl and reserve the liquid.
8. Carefully remove the meat from the bones after letting it cool for some time.
9. Shred the boneless chicken with two forks and add cooking liquid over it to moisten (don't pour all the liquid, add only what is required).
10. You can then strain the remaining liquid and use it as chicken stock.
11. Transfer the moistened meat over the plate. Sprinkle black pepper if you want it hot.
12. Serve immediately and enjoy!

Arianna Brooks

Slow-Cooker Chicken Parmesan Meatballs

Makes: 10 servings

Carbs per serving: 7 grams

Ingredients:

For the meatballs

- 1 pound chicken (ground)
- 30 fresh mozzarella balls (pearl-size)
- 1/2 cup fine dry breadcrumbs (whole-wheat)
- 1 lightly beaten large egg
- 1/2 teaspoon dried oregano
- 1/2 cup Parmesan cheese (grated)
- 1/2 teaspoon basil (dried)
- 1/4 teaspoon salt
- 1/2 teaspoon garlic powder
- Chopped parsley or spring onions (for garnishing)

For the sauce

- 1/2 medium onion (grated)
- 28 ounces unsalted crushed tomatoes (1 can)
- 2 minced garlic cloves
- 1/4 cup dry red wine
- 1/2 teaspoon dried oregano
- 1/4 teaspoon salt
- 1/2 teaspoon dried basil

Instructions:

1. Combine the onion, tomatoes, garlic, red wine, oregano, salt and basil in the slow cooker to prepare the sauce. Set aside.
2. Take a medium bowl and place the ground chicken in it.
3. Add the beaten egg, breadcrumbs, oregano, Parmesan cheese, salt and garlic powder to the chicken in the bowl.
4. Mix well until the contents are well combined and you get a thick dough consistency.
5. Take 1 tablespoon of the seasoned meat and pat it on a disk. Place a mozzarella ball in the center and wrap the meat around as you roll it into a ball.
6. Repeat step 5 with the remaining meat mixture and keep them ready
7. Add these meatballs to the sauce mixture in the slow cooker.
8. Cover the cooker and cook on high for 3 hours or cook on low heat for 6 hours
9. Once the cooking cycle is over, transfer the meatballs to the serving plate.
10. Pour the thick sauce from the cooker over the meatballs and sprinkle some chopped parsley or spring onions over it.
11. Serve warm and enjoy!

Arianna Brooks

Wine & Tomato Braised Chicken

Makes: 10 servings

Carbs per serving: 5 grams

Ingredients:

- 1 cup dry white wine
- 28 ounces coarsely chopped whole tomatoes with juice (1 can)
- 10 skinless trimmed bone-in chicken thighs (about 3 3/4 pounds),
- 4 bacon slices
- 1/4 cup fresh parsley (finely chopped)
- 1 finely chopped large onion
- 1 teaspoon pepper (freshly ground)
- 4 minced garlic cloves
- 1 teaspoon fennel seeds
- 1 teaspoon dried thyme
- 1 teaspoon salt
- 1 bay leaf
- Nonstick cooking spray

Instructions:

1. Grease a large skillet with nonstick cooking spray and heat it over medium heat.
2. Place the bacon slices on the hot skillet and cook for 4 minutes until they become crisp.
3. Transfer the crisp bacon to paper towels and let it drain. When it cools, crumble them well.
4. The skillet will have the fat from the cooked bacon; drain them off leaving only 2 tablespoons of the fat.

5. Add onion to the skillet and cook in the fat over medium heat for 6 minutes until tender. Stir often.
6. Add the bay leaf, dried thyme, fennel seeds, garlic cloves and pepper to the onion in the skillet.
7. Continue to cook for a minute as you stir the mixture. Add the wine and bring it to boil for 2 minutes. Scrape up the browned bits from the bottom or sides of the skillet.
8. Now add the tomatoes along with their juice. Season with salt and stir well until combined.
9. Take a slow cooker and place the chicken thighs into it. Sprinkle the crumbled bacon over it.
10. Pour the tomato mixture over the chicken and cover the cooker.
11. Cook on high for 3 hours or on low heat for 6 hours until the chicken is completely cooked and tender.
12. Remove the bay leaf and transfer to a plate.
13. Sprinkle the chopped parsley and serve warm!

Arianna Brooks

Chicken and Pepperoni

Makes: 6 servings

Carbs per serving: 1 gram

Ingredients:

- 4 pounds skinless meaty chicken pieces (drumsticks, breast halves, and thighs)
- 2 ounces turkey pepperoni (sliced)
- 1/2 cup reduced-sodium chicken broth
- 1/4 cup ripe olives (sliced and pitted)
- 1 tablespoon tomato paste
- 1/2 cup part-skim mozzarella cheese (shredded) – about 2 ounces should do
- 1/8 teaspoon salt
- 1 teaspoon crushed dried Italian seasoning
- 1/8 teaspoon black pepper (ground)
- Nonstick cooking spray

Instructions:

1. Grease the insides of the slow cooker with a nonstick cooking spray.
2. Place the chicken pieces in the slow cooker. Sprinkle pepper and salt over the pieces. Toss it once.
3. Cut the sliced pepperoni into half and add it to the cooker. Also add the olives to the contents in the cooker and set aside.
4. Take a small bowl and combine the tomato paste, chicken broth and Italian seasoning together. Whisk the contents together until blended well.

5. Add this mixture to the contents of the cooker and cover.
6. Cook on high for 3.5 hours and on low heat for 7 hours
7. Transfer the pepperoni, chicken and olives to a plate using a slotted spoon. Discard the liquid in the cooker.
8. Sprinkle the cheese over the contents (pepperoni-chicken-olive) in the plate.
9. Loosely cover the plate with an aluminum foil and let it sit for 5 minutes until the cheese melts.
10. Serve warm and enjoy!

Arianna Brooks

Barbecue Pulled Chicken

Makes: 8 servings

Carbs per serving: 9 grams

Ingredients:

- 2 1/2 pounds fat-trimmed chicken thighs (boneless and skinless)
- 1 finely chopped small onion
- 4 ounces chopped and drained green chilies (1 can)
- 1 minced garlic clove
- 8 ounces reduced-sodium tomato sauce (1 can)
- 3 tablespoons apple cider vinegar
- 1 tablespoon Worcestershire sauce
- 2 tablespoons honey
- 2 teaspoons dry mustard
- 1 tablespoon smoked or sweet paprika
- 1 teaspoon ground chipotle chili
- 1 tablespoon tomato paste
- 1/2 teaspoon salt

Instructions:

1. Combine the tomato paste, ground chipotle, salt, paprika, mustard, honey, Worcestershire sauce, apple cider vinegar and tomato sauce in the slow cooker.
2. Mix them well until smooth and the flavors get blended.
3. Add the onion and garlic to this sauce mixture. Stir the contents once more before you add the chicken to the cooker.
4. Stir the entire contents thoroughly until the ingredients are well incorporated.

5. Cover the cooker and cook on high for 3 hours and on low heat for 5 hours
6. After the cooking cycle, transfer the cooked chicken to a clean cutting board. Shred the meat with two forks.
7. Add the shredded meat back to the slow cooker and stir it well until the sauce and chicken pieces combine.
8. Transfer to a plate and serve warm.

Arianna Brooks

Asian Style Slow Cooked Chicken Wings

Makes: 2 servings

Carbs per serving: 4 grams

Ingredients:

- 1.5 pounds of raw chicken wings prepared
- 1 teaspoon red pepper flakes
- 1/4 cup soy sauce
- 1 teaspoon garlic paste
- 2 tablespoons lime juice
- Sliced green onions, chopped fresh cilantro, lime wedges - for garnishing
- Salt and black pepper, to taste
- 1 teaspoon low carb sweetener
- Nonstick cooking spray

Instructions:

1. Grease the inside of the slow cooker with nonstick cooking spray.
2. Place the prepared chicken wings in the cooker and set aside.
3. Take a small bowl and combine together the red pepper flakes, soy sauce, garlic paste and lime juice.
4. Pour this mixture over the chicken wings in the cooker and close the lid.
5. Cook on high for 2.5 hours until the wings are thoroughly cooked and tender
6. Line a baking sheet with parchment paper and place the cooked wings.

7. Season with pepper and salt. Broil for 10 minutes until the wings turn crisp.
8. Transfer to plate and garnish with green onions, fresh cilantro and lime wedges.
9. Serve warm and enjoy!

Arianna Brooks

Italian Chicken

Makes: 3 servings

Carbs per serving: 1 gram

Ingredients:

- 1 1/2 lb. chicken pieces
- 1/8 cup melted unsalted butter
- 1/2 Tbsp. lemon juice
- 1/2 Tbsp. oregano
- A dash each of: dried oregano, onion powder, dried basil, paprika, black pepper, garlic powder, granulated sugar

Instructions:

1. Put the chicken pieces inside the slow cooker.
2. In a bowl, combine the melted butter, lemon juice, and seasonings. Pour this all over the chicken.
3. Cover and cook for 4 hours on high or until the chicken is well done. Toss in the sauce to coat and sprinkle with oregano an hour before the end of cooking time.

Chicken in Wine Sauce

Makes: 4 servings

Carbs per serving: 4 grams

Ingredients:

- 1 lb. chicken breasts
- 5 oz. low sodium cream of mushroom soup
- 1 Tbsp. low sodium onion soup mix
- 1/2 cup dry white wine

Instructions:

1. Arrange the chicken breasts in the slow cooker.
2. In a bowl, mix together the rest of the ingredients and pour the mixture on top of the chicken.
3. Cover and cook for 6 hours on low or until chicken becomes well done.

Arianna Brooks

Thai Chicken

Makes: 3 servings

Carbs per serving: 7 grams

Ingredients:

- 3 skinless chicken thighs
- 1/3 cup low sodium salsa
- 1/4 cup chunky peanut butter
- 1 Tbsp. lime juice
- 1/2 Tbsp. low sodium soy sauce
- 1/2 tsp grated fresh ginger
- 1/2 Tbsp. chopped cilantro

Instructions:

1. Arrange the chicken thighs in the slow cooker.
2. In a bowl, combine the rest of the ingredients, except the cilantro. Pour the mixture all over the chicken thighs.
3. Cover and cook for 8 hours on low, or until the chicken is well done. Remove any fat, then transfer the chicken onto a serving plate.
4. Spoon the sauce on top of the chicken and top with cilantro.

Curried Chicken with Tomatoes

Makes: 3 servings

Carbs per serving: 13 grams

Ingredients:

- 14 oz. unsalted diced tomatoes
- 2 boneless and skinless chicken breasts, sliced in half
- 1/2 cup coarsely chopped onion
- 1/4 cup chopped carrots
- 1/4 cup chopped green bell pepper
- 1/4 cup chopped celery
- 1/2 tsp turmeric
- 1 Tbsp. curry powder
- 1/8 tsp black pepper
- 1/2 Tbsp. brown sugar

Instructions:

1. Mix together all of the ingredients in the slow cooker.
2. Cover and cook for 5 hours on low or for 2 hours on high, or until the chicken is well done.

Arianna Brooks

Oriental Ginger Chicken

Makes: 3 servings

Carbs per serving: 8 grams

Ingredients:

- 3 boneless and skinless chicken breasts, cubed
- 1/2 cup diced carrots
- 1/4 cup low sodium soy sauce
- 1/8 cup chopped onion
- 1/8 cup rice vinegar
- 1/2 Tbsp. ground ginger
- 1/8 cup sesame seeds
- 1/2 tsp sesame oil
- 1/2 cup cauliflower
- 1/2 cup broccoli

Instructions:

1. Brown the chicken breasts in a greased skillet over medium high flame, then transfer into the slow cooker.
2. Add the rest of the ingredients, except the cauliflower and broccoli, into the slow cooker. Cover and cook for 4 hours on low.
3. Add the cauliflower and broccoli and mix well. Cook for an additional hour, then serve.

Stuffed Chicken Breast

Makes: 4 servings

Carbs per serving: 0 grams

Ingredients:

- 2 boneless and skinless chicken breasts
- 4 slices Swiss cheese
- 4 slices low sodium bacon
- 1/6 cup low sodium chicken broth
- 1/3 cup white cooking wine
- Black pepper

Instructions:

1. Slice each breast in half, lengthwise, then flatten until half an inch thick.
2. Put a slice of cheese over each breast, then season with black pepper. Roll up and wrap a strip of bacon around each. Lock everything in place using a toothpick.
3. Arrange the stuffed chicken breasts in the slow cooker.
4. In a bowl, mix together the wine and broth, then pour this into the slow cooker. Cover and cook for 4 hours on high.

Arianna Brooks

Roast Turkey Breast

Makes: 3 servings

Carbs per serving: 0 grams

Ingredients:

- 1/2 turkey breast
- 1/2 Tbsp. dried minced onion
- 1/2 tsp no sodium beef bouillon
- 1/4 tsp onion powder
- 1/16 tsp black pepper
- 1/16 tsp paprika

Instructions:

1. In a bowl, mix together the onion, beef bouillon, onion powder, black pepper, and paprika.
2. Wash and rinse the turkey breast very well. Pat dry using kitchen paper towels. Rub the onion mixture all over the chicken breast.
3. Place the chicken breast inside the slow cooker. Cover and cook for 45 minutes on high, then reduce setting to low and cook for 5 hours.

Chicken Parmesan

Makes: 3 servings

Carbs per serving: 12.8 g

Ingredients:

- ¾ pound boneless, skinless chicken breast, cut into serving size pieces
- 14 ounce can crushed tomatoes
- 2 cloves garlic, minced
- ½ a 4 ounce can sliced black olives (optional)
- 2 ounce sliced mushrooms
- 1 teaspoon oregano
- 1 teaspoon basil
- ½ teaspoon thyme
- 3 ounce mozzarella cheese

Instructions:

1. Mix together in a bowl all the ingredients except the chicken and mozzarella.
2. Place the chicken in the slow cooker.
3. Cover and cook on low for 8 hours or until done.
4. Place an ounce of mozzarella over each chicken piece a couple of minutes before serving.
5. Serve when the cheese melts.

Arianna Brooks

Olive Oil and Rosemary Chicken

Makes: 8 servings

Carbs per serving: 1.4 grams

Ingredients:

- 8 cloves of garlic, sliced
- ½ tsp of kosher salt
- 1 tbsp. of dried rosemary, crumble using your fingers
- ½ tsp of black pepper
- 3 tbsp. of white wine
- 3 tbsp. of extra-virgin olive oil
- 2 tbsp. of water
- 2 lbs. of boneless and skinless chicken breasts
- Cooking spray

Instructions:

1. Lightly cover the slow cooker with cooking spray. Add in the garlic, rosemary, kosher salt, black pepper, extra-virgin olive oil, white wine and water into the slow cooker and mix well.
2. Place the chicken into the Crockpot one at a time and make sure to cover each piece with sauce.
3. Cook for 8 hours on low setting or 4 hours on high.

Cheesy Chicken

Makes: 4 servings

Carbs per serving: 9.5 grams

Ingredients:

- 4 halves of skinless and boneless chicken breast
- 18 oz. of cream cheese (reduced-fat)
- 1 can of cream of mushroom soup
- 1.5 cups of water
- 1 pack of Italian dressing mix

Instructions:

1. Place the chicken inside the slow cooker.
2. Combine water and Italian dressing mix and pour it over the chicken.
3. Cook the chicken for 4 hours over low setting. An hour before serving, remove the chicken from the slow cooker and shred using a fork. Place the chicken into the Crockpot again and add in the cream of mushroom and cream cheese. Combine well.

Arianna Brooks

Salsa Chicken

Makes: 10 servings

Carbs per serving: 3.9 grams

Ingredients:

- 5 pieces of chicken breasts
- ½ pack of taco seasoning
- 16 oz. of La Victoria mild salsa (Thick 'N Chunky)

Instructions:

1. Remove the excess fat from the chicken. Rinse the meat and place it inside the slow cooker.
2. Sprinkle the taco seasoning on the chicken. Pour in the salsa over the meat.
3. Cook for 8 hours on low settings.

Neufchatel Chicken

Makes: 16 servings

Carbs per serving: 3.1 grams

Ingredients:

- 3 lbs. of skinless and boneless chicken
- Cooking spray
- ¼ cup of Italian dressing
- 1 small onion, chopped
- 1 can of cream of chicken soup
- 1 clove of garlic, chopped
- 8 oz. of Neufchatel cheese
- ½ cup of chicken broth (reduced-sodium)

Instructions:

1. Place the chicken meat into the slow cooker and coat the meat with Italian dressing.
2. Cook for 6 hours on low setting.
3. Meanwhile, lightly coat a medium saucepan with cooking spray and cook the garlic and onion for 2 minutes. Add in the chicken broth, cream of chicken soup and Neufchatel cheese. Stir until the mixture is consistent.
4. Once the chicken is cooked, add in the contents of the saucepan into the slow cooker and cook for another hour.

Arianna Brooks

Lemon Chicken

Makes: 8 servings

Carbs per serving: 1.6 grams

Ingredients:

- 1 tsp of dried oregano
- ¼ tsp of pepper
- ½ tsp of salt
- 2 lbs. of skinless and boneless chicken tenders
- ½ cup of chicken broth
- 2 tbsp. of butter substitute
- ½ cup of white wine
- 2 cloves of garlic, minced
- 1/3 cup of fresh lemon juice
- 1 tsp of chicken bouillon granules
- ½ tsp of dried parsley

Instructions:

1. Prepare a saucepan. Add in the oregano, salt, pepper, butter substitute, chicken broth, white wine, lemon juice, garlic, chicken bouillon and dried parsley. Mix well and bring the mixture to a boil.
2. Place the chicken meat into the Crockpot and pour the mixture on top.
3. Cook for 3 hours on low setting.

Vegetable and Herbed Chicken Stew

Makes: 6 servings

Carbs per serving: 13.5 grams

Ingredients:

- 2 cups of culinary broth (white wine and herb)
- 1 ½ cup of diced potato
- 1 cup of chopped carrots
- 1 cup of diced celery
- ½ cup of tomato sauce (no salt added)
- 1 medium onion
- 2 cups of water
- 1 ½ tsp of red pepper
- 28 oz. of skinless chicken breast
- ½ tsp of dried marjoram
- ¼ tsp of chili powder
- ½ tsp of black pepper
- ½ tbsp. of basil
- 3 cloves of garlic

Instructions:

1. Place the chicken meat inside the slow cooker. Add in the broth, carrots, potato, celery, onion, tomato sauce, water, red pepper, marjoram, black pepper, chili powder, basil and garlic. Mix well.
2. Cook for 8 hours on low setting or 4 hours on high.

Arianna Brooks

Thai Green Chicken Curry

Makes: 4 servings

Carbs per serving: 5.9 grams

Ingredients:

- ¾ can light coconut milk
- 1 ½ tablespoon green curry paste
- 1 ½ tablespoon brown sugar
- 3 cloves garlic, minced
- 1 ¼ pound chicken breast, cut into small chunks
- ½ a bag stir fry fresh vegetables of your choice
- ½ a can baby corn, drained
- 1 medium red onion, sliced
- 1 tablespoon cornstarch
- 2 tablespoons water

Instructions:

- Add coconut milk, curry paste, brown sugar, and garlic to the pot of the slow cooker. Whisk well.
- Add rest of the ingredients except cornstarch and water.
- Cover and cook on low for 5 hours.
- Mix together cornstarch and water and add to the pot. Mix well. Just in case you like your vegetables to be crunchy, then add the vegetables now instead of earlier.
- Cover and cook for 30 minutes or until the curry becomes thick.
- Serve hot with cauliflower rice.

Note: The carbs value does not include cauliflower rice.

Gourmet Chicken

Makes: 7 servings

Carbs per serving: 11.6 grams

Ingredients:

- 1 cup of wild rice
- 1 pack of frozen cauliflower
- 14 oz. of skinless chicken breast
- ½ pack of frozen broccoli
- 1 can of cream of celery soup
- 3 tbsp. of light dressing
- 1 ½ cans of hot water

Instructions:

1. Add in the wild rice into the slow cooker. Add in the cauliflower and broccoli.
2. Add in the light dressing and cream of celery soup. The chicken breast should be added next.
3. Cook for 7 hours on low setting. Give it a quick stir after the first 4 hours of cooking time.

Arianna Brooks

Orange Chicken

Makes: 4 servings

Carbs per serving: 1.1 grams

Ingredients:

- 4 green onions, sliced
- 1 tbsp. of black sesame seeds
- 1 ½lbs of chicken legs
- ¼ tsp. of fish sauce
- ½ tsp. of orange oil
- ½ tsp. of toasted sesame seeds
- ½ tsp. of freshly grated ginger
- 1 tsp. of coconut aminos
- 1 tsp. of toasted sesame oil
- 2 tbsp. of Swerve Confectioners
- ¼ cup of coconut milk
- ¼ cup of melted coconut oil

Instructions:

1. In a mixing bowl, combine the fish sauce, orange oil, toasted sesame seeds, ginger, coconut aminos, sesame oil, Swerve Confectioners, coconut milk, and coconut oil. Whisk the ingredients together until well incorporated.
2. Place the chicken meat into the slow cooker and pour the sauce over the meat.
3. Cover and cook for 8 hours on low settings.

Indian Butter Chicken

Makes: 3 servings

Carbs per serving: 5.1 grams

Ingredients:

- 1 pound chicken breasts, cubed
- ½ tablespoon vegetable oil
- 1 shallot, finely chopped
- 1 onion, chopped
- 1 tablespoon butter
- 1 teaspoon lemon juice
- 2 cloves garlic, minced
- ½ inch piece ginger, minced
- 1 teaspoon garam masala (Indian spice blend)
- ½ teaspoon chili powder
- ½ teaspoon ground cumin
- 1 bay leaf
- 2 tablespoons plain non fat yogurt
- 2 tablespoons half and half
- 6 tablespoons skim milk
- ½ cup tomato sauce
- 1 teaspoon cayenne pepper or to taste
- Salt to taste
- 1/8 teaspoon pepper powder
- Cilantro leaves for garnishing

Instructions:

1. Place a skillet over medium heat. Add oil. When oil is heated, add onions and shallot and sauté until translucent.

2. Add ginger and garlic and sauté for a couple of minutes. Add garam masala, cumin, cayenne, chili powder, and bay leaf. Sauté for a few seconds. Add tomato sauce, milk, half and half and yogurt. Lower heat and simmer for 5-6 minutes. Stir on and off.
3. Remove from heat. Add salt and pepper. Cool slightly and blend in a blender or with a stick blender until smooth
4. Add the chicken pieces to the slow cooker. Pour the blended mixture to the cooker. Mix well.
5. Cover and cook for 4 hours on low or until done.
6. Garnish with cilantro leaves and serve hot with cauliflower rice.

Note: The carbs value does not include the cauliflower rice.

Mediterranean Roast Turkey

Makes: 4 servings

Carbs per serving: 7 grams

Ingredients

- 1 cup chopped onions
- ¼ cup kalamata olives, pitted
- ¼ cup julienne cut drained oil packed sun dried tomato halves
- 1 tablespoon fresh lemon juice
- 1 teaspoon garlic, minced
- 1 teaspoon Greek seasoning mix
- ½ teaspoon salt or to taste
- Freshly ground black pepper to taste
- 2 pounds boneless turkey breast, trimmed
- ½ cup fat free low sodium chicken broth, divided
- 1 ½ tablespoons all-purpose flour
- Thyme sprigs (optional)

Instructions:

1. Add all the ingredients except broth, flour, and thyme to the slow cooker.
2. Add half the broth. Cover and cook on low for 7 hours.
3. In a small bowl, mix together the remaining broth and flour. Mix well until smooth. Add this to the cooker. Stir well. Cover and cook for 30 minutes more until the sauce thickens.
4. Slice the turkey and serve with the sauce.

Arianna Brooks

Asian Braised Turkey with Vegetables

Makes: 4 servings

Carbs per serving: 11.3 grams

Ingredients:

- 1 package (3 ½ ounce) shiitake mushrooms, remove stems, slice
- ½ cup thinly sliced red bell pepper
- 3 baby bok choy, quartered lengthwise
- 3 bamboo shoots, sliced
- ½ a 15 ounce can precut baby corn, drained
- 1 tablespoon Hoisin sauce
- 1 tablespoon oyster sauce
- ½ tablespoon low sodium soy sauce
- 1 teaspoon fresh grated ginger
- 1 teaspoon dark sesame oil
- 2 cloves garlic, minced
- ½ tablespoon canola oil
- 2 pounds bone-in turkey thighs, skinned
- ½ teaspoon 5 spice powder
- ¼ teaspoon freshly ground pepper
- 1 cup thinly sliced Napa cabbage
- ¼ cup chopped green onions

Instructions:

1. Place a nonstick pan over medium heat. Add canola oil and heat. Meanwhile season the turkey thighs with 5-spice powder and pepper. Add the turkey to the pan. If the quantity is too much for your pan, then do it in

batches. Brown the turkey on both the sides until browned.
2. Add mushrooms, bell pepper, bok choy, baby corn, and bamboo shoots to the slow cooker.
3. Add the browned turkey to the cooker.
4. Mix together in a bowl, all the sauces, ginger, garlic, and sesame oil. Pour this over the vegetables in the cooker.
5. Cover and cook on low for 5 hours or until the turkey is done.
6. Separate the turkey from the bones and discard the bones. Cut the turkey into bite size pieces.
7. To the cooker, add cabbage and mix well.
8. Pour into individual bowls. Place the chopped turkey over the vegetables and sprinkle with green onions.

Arianna Brooks

Jamaican Jerk Chicken

Makes: 4 servings

Carbs per serving: 1.8 grams

Ingredients:

- ¾ pound boneless, skinless chicken thighs
- ¾ pound bone-in skinless chicken breasts
- 2 tablespoons fresh lime juice
- 2 cloves garlic
- 1 tablespoon fresh thyme
- ½ tablespoon fresh ginger, grated
- ½ tablespoon dark brown sugar
- 1 teaspoon allspice berries
- 2 scallions, sliced
- 2 habanero peppers or to taste
- ¾ teaspoon salt or to taste
- Pepper powder to taste
- 1 tablespoon white vinegar
- 2 tablespoons water
- ½ red pepper

Instructions:

1. Blend together all the ingredients except the chicken to a smooth paste.
2. Add the chicken to the slow cooker. Pour the blended ingredients over the chicken.
3. Cover and cook on low for 6 hours or until done.

Spicy Chicken Drumsticks

Makes: 2 servings

Carbs per serving: 3 grams

Ingredients:

- 1 lb. chicken drumsticks (4 pcs), skinned
- 1/2 cup of bottled picante sauce
- 1/8 tsp cayenne pepper or 2 tsp of bottled cayenne pepper sauce or
- 1/2 tsp smoked paprika
- 1/4 tsp dried thyme, crushed
- 1 bay leaf
- 2 tsp olive oil

Instructions:

1. Get your slow cooker and lightly coat it with cooking spray. Put the chicken at the bottom. Combine the pepper sauce, picante sauce, thyme, paprika, and bay leaf in a small bowl. Spoon the chicken over to the slow cooker.
2. Cover the pot and allow to cook for 6 hours on low heat or for about 3 hours on high.
3. Remove the chicken pieces and transfer to a serving dish. Get rid of the bay leaf from thee sauce in the cooker, then stir the oil in. Spoon the sauce over the chicken evenly. Put a cover and set aside for about 10 minutes to let the chicken absorb all the flavors.
4. Pour around 1 tsp of sauce over each of the drumsticks. Take the remaining sauce away.
5. Serve immediately.

Arianna Brooks

Greek-Style Stuffed Chicken Breasts

Makes: 6 servings

Carbs per serving: 4.3 grams

Ingredients:

- 2 lbs. skinless boneless chicken breasts
- 3 cups spinach, finely chopped
- 2 red peppers, roasted and chopped
- 1/4 cup black olives, sliced
- 1 tbsp. oregano, chopped
- 1 cup artichoke hearts, chopped
- 4 ounces reduced fat feta
- 1 tsp. garlic powder
- 1.5 cups chicken broth
- Salt & pepper

Instructions:

1. Get a bowl and combine together the spinach, feta, artichoke hearts, roasted red peppers, garlic, and oregano.
2. Season the chicken breasts with salt & pepper.
3. Using a sharp knife, cut deep into the core of the chicken breasts, creating a pocket. Avoid cutting through the meat.
4. Get the spinach mixture and stuff the chicken breasts.
5. Put everything into the slow cooker. To make sure that all the chicken fits, you may need to slowly put them on their side. The spinach mixture is placed facing up, stacked sideways along the slow cooker's bottom. This

way, you prevent the stuffing from getting loose and falling out.
6. Place the chicken both.
7. Allow to cook for about 4 hours. Check from time to time to make sure that the chicken breasts are completely cooked through.

Arianna Brooks

Buffalo Chicken

Makes: 6 servings

Carbs per serving: 8.1 grams

Ingredients:

- 2 lbs. skinless, boneless chicken
- 2 pcs. whole carrots
- 2 pcs. Whole ribs celery
- 1 small-sized onion, quartered
- 2 clove garlic
- 1 ½ cups of chicken broth
- Salt & pepper
- ½ to 2/3 cup of buffalo sauce
- 2 tbsp. of butter, more for additional servings (optional)

Instructions:

1. Place the chicken, celery ribs, whole garlic and cloves, onion, carrots, and chicken broth inside the slow cooker. Add salt & pepper to season.
2. Allow to cook for about 4 hours on high heat setting. Discard the cooking liquid, retaining only 1/3 cup with the veggies. Using 2 forks shred the chicken meat.
3. Pour the buffalo sauce and butter (optional). Allow to cook for another 15 minutes.

Slow Cooker Low Carb

Butter Chicken Special

Makes: 6 servings

Carbs per serving: 5.1 grams

Ingredients:

- 2 lbs. of chicken breast, cubed
- 1 shallot, chopped finely
- 1 tbsp. vegetable oil
- 1/4 white onion, chopped
- 2 tbsp. butter
- 2 tsp lemon juice
- 4 cloves garlic, minced
- 1 inch-long ginger, minced
- 2 tsp of garam masala
- 1 tsp of chili powder
- 1 tsp of ground cumin
- 1 pc bay leaf
- 1/4 cup of non-fat yogurt, plain
- 3/4 cup of skim milk
- 1/4 cup of half and half milk
- 1 cup of tomato sauce
- 2 1/4 tsp cayenne pepper, to taste
- 1 pinch of salt
- 1 pinch of black pepper

Instructions:

1. Get a medium-sized saucepan and heat oil on medium heat setting. Put the onion and shallot in, and sauté until tender.

2. Add the lemon juice, butter, garlic, ginger, chili powder, garam masala, cumin, bay leaf, and cayenne. Cook for about 1 minute or just enough until you smell the fragrance.
3. Put the tomato sauce into the mix; cook for 2 more minutes, frequently stirring.
4. Add the skim milk, half and half, and yogurt. Adjust the heat to low, simmer as you stir, for about 10 minutes. Stir continuously.
5. Season with some salt & pepper, as necessary.
6. Put everything in a blender and process until combined well.
7. Put the chicken breast cubes in the crockpot and allow to cook for about 4 hours.
8. Best served with cauliflower rice or plain rice.

Slow Cooker Low Carb

Pollo Pibil

Makes: 8 servings

Carbs per serving: 3.8 grams

Ingredients:

- 3 lbs. skinless, boneless, chicken thighs, fat trimmed
- 1/2 cup of orange juice
- 2 pcs. Habaneros, seeded & diced
- 3 cloves garlic, diced
- 1 pc onion, cut into quarters
- 1 tbsp. of coriander
- 1 tsp of cumin
- 1 tsp of dried oregano
- 4 tbsp. of Achiote paste
- 1/4 cup of chicken broth
- Salt & pepper
- 1/2 cup apple cider vinegar

Instructions:

1. Season the chicken thighs with salt & pepper, and then place in the slow cooker.
2. Put the rest of the ingredients in a blender, and process to create the sauce. Pour the sauce into the crockpot, on top of the chicken.
3. Cook for about 4 hours on low heat setting or until the chicken is tender enough to be easily shredded using 2 forks.
4. Shred the meat, then continue to cook for 30 minutes more, with the cooker cover off. This will help thicken the sauce a bit.
5. Take the chicken out of the cooker.

6. Serve with burritos, tacos, rice, or on its own. It can also be served as tostadas over oven-baked tortillas. If preferred, garnish with red onion pickles.
7. Enjoy while hot.

Chicken Barbacoa

Makes: 6 servings

Carbs per serving: 4.3 grams

Ingredients:

- 2 lbs. chicken breasts
- 1/2 can (17 oz.) of chipotles in adobo sauce
- 1 pc onion, quartered
- 4 whole garlic cloves
- 1/2 tbsp. of cumin
- 1 tsp. of oregano
- 1/2 cup of chicken broth
- Salt & pepper

Instructions:

1. First, season the chicken breasts with salt & pepper. Put it inside the slow cooker together with the garlic cloves and onion.
2. Put the chipotles, oregano, cumin, and chicken broth in slow cooker and stir to blend the ingredients together.
3. Allow to cook for about 4 hours over high heat. Once done, take the garlic, onions, and chipotles out.
4. Shred the chicken with 2 forks.
5. Transfer to a serving dish and serve while hot.

Arianna Brooks

Eggplant Turkey Bolognese

Makes: 8 servings

Carbs per serving: 8 grams

Ingredients:

- 1 lb. lean turkey, ground
- 1 onion, diced
- 4 to 6 cloves of garlic, minced
- 3/4 tsp of salt
- 1/2 tsp of pepper
- 1 ½ lbs. eggplant, 1 large eggplant, chopped (about 8 cups)
- 1/2 cup of chicken broth
- 1 can (28 oz.) of whole tomatoes
- 1/2 cup of parmesan cheese
- 1-2 pcs of bay leaves

Instructions:

1. Get a non-stick skillet and heat on medium high setting. Put the meat, onion, garlic, and salt & pepper. Cook until browned or for around 10 minutes.
2. Put the browned turkey meat into the slow cooker. Add the rest of the ingredients. Stir and combine well.
3. Allow to cook for about 6 to 8 hours on low heat setting or until the eggplant is completely broken down.

Roasted Sticky Chicken

Makes: 8 servings

Carbs per serving: 1.7 grams

Ingredients:

- 1 roasting chicken, whole
- 1 tsp of paprika
- 1/2 tsp of onion powder
- 1 tsp of pepper
- 1 tsp of cayenne pepper
- 1 tsp of garlic powder
- 1 pc small onion, chopped

Instructions:

1. Put the chicken together with the dry ingredients inside a gallon-sized ziplock bag. Refrigerate overnight. Dump the bag's contents into the slow cooker the following day.
2. Set the cooker to low heat and cook for about 8 to 10 hours. Once done, carefully extract the chicken from the cooker as it falls apart because of its tenderness.
3. Serve with Bulgar, couscous, or rice.

Arianna Brooks

Marinara Chicken & Veggies

Makes: 8 servings

Carbs per serving: 7.9 grams

Ingredients:

- 2 lbs. skinless, boneless chicken breasts
- 4 cloves of garlic, peeled & crushed
- 4 pcs tomatoes, chopped
- 4 medium-sized ribs celery, diced
- 2 small-sized zucchinis, diced
- 1 pc bell pepper, cored, seeded, & diced
- 1 jar (18 oz.) of low-sodium marinara sauce
- 1 tsp of dried basil
- 1 tsp of dried thyme

Instructions:

1. Carefully set the chicken inside the crockpot, then add the tomatoes, celery, garlic, pepper, and zucchinis. Scatter the marinara sauce over the ingredients, and drizzle the top with thyme and basil.
2. Cook for about 6 to 7 hours on low heat setting.
3. Shred the chicken while still inside the crockpot using a fork. Transfer the contents of the cooker to a serving dish.
4. Serve and enjoy while hot.

Mustard Honey Turkey Stew

Makes: 6 servings

Carbs per serving: 14 grams

Ingredients:

- 1 cup of carrots, chopped
- 1 ½ cups of celery, chopped
- 1 ½ cups of onions, chopped
- 1 cup of unsalted chicken broth
- 2 tbsp. of honey
- 1 tsp of rosemary, dried
- 2 tbsp. of grainy Dijon mustard
- 1 large-sized turkey breast, chunked
- 2 tbsp. of spelt flour (or brown rice flour, oat or whole wheat flour)

Instructions:

1. Toss the turkey chunks in flour for coating. Put all the ingredients in the slow cooker. Stir and cover.
2. Allow to cook for about 6 to 8 hours on low heat setting, or 3 to 4 hours on high.
3. Serve and enjoy.

Arianna Brooks

Chicken Gyros

Makes: 8 servings

Carbs per serving: 10 grams

Ingredients:

For the Main Dish

- 1/2 pc small onion
- 3 cloves of garlic
- 2 lbs. of ground chicken
- 2 eggs, whisked
- 1/2 cup of whole wheat bread crumbs, plain
- 1 pc lemon, juiced & zested
- 1 tsp of dried thyme
- 1/4 tsp of cinnamon
- 1/4 tsp of nutmeg
- 2 tsp of salt
- 1 tbsp. of extra virgin olive oil
- 12 mini-sized whole wheat naan

For the Toppings

- 1 pc tomato, chopped
- 1/2 cup of plain Greek yogurt, low fat
- 1 cucumber, sliced
- 1 lemon, sliced into wedges

Instructions:

1. Pulse the garlic and onion and puree using a food processor.

2. Get a large-sized bowl and mix the ground chicken, onion puree, breadcrumbs, eggs, lemon zest and juice, cinnamon, thyme, salt, and nutmeg together. Stir until everything is well combined.
3. Shape the mixture into 1 large ball, and then put it in the slow cooker that has been sprinkled with some olive oil.
4. Allow to cook for about 4 to 6 hours over high heat setting or 6 to 8 hours on low.
5. Turn the heat off and take the lid off about half an hour prior to serving the dish. This will provide sufficient time for the dish to set.
6. Once ready to serve. Take the meat out of the crockpot and slice.
7. Best served on warm pita bread with toppings of cucumber, yogurt, tomato, and juice from a freshly squeezed lemon.

Arianna Brooks

Chicken Marsala

Makes: 12 servings

Carbs per serving: 9.4 grams

Ingredients:
- 6 pcs skinless, boneless, chicken breasts,
- 2 cloves garlic, minced
- 2 tbsp. of extra virgin olive oil
- 1 tsp of salt
- 1 tsp of pepper
- 2 cups of chicken broth or Marsala wine
- 1 Cup cold water
- 1/2 cup of arrowroot powder
- 16 oz. of baby Portobello mushrooms, sliced
- 3 tbsp. of parsley, fresh chopped

Instructions:
1. Halve the chicken breasts length-wise then set aside.
2. Grease the slow cooker then put the oil and garlic.
3. Season the chicken breasts with salt & pepper on both sides and gently place in the slow cooker.
4. Pour the wine on the chicken then cover the cooker.
5. Allow to cook for 3 hours on high, or 7 hours on low heat setting.
6. Combine the arrowroot with water and stir continuously until there are no more lumps.
7. Take the chicken out of the cooker and keep it warm.
8. Put the arrowroot mixture at the bottom of the cooker and add the mushrooms.

9. Put the chicken back in, and stir the mushrooms and sauce to fully coat the chicken.
10. Cover the crockpot and cook for another hour.
11. Drizzle with freshly chopped parsley and serve.

Arianna Brooks

Slow Cooker Turkey Breast with Gravy

Makes: 5 servings

Carbs per serving: 8 grams

Ingredients:

- ¾ tablespoon unsalted butter or olive oil
- 1 medium carrot, peeled, chopped
- 3 cloves garlic, peeled, crushed
- 1 cup low sodium chicken broth
- 2 tablespoons dry white wine
- 1 bay leaf
- 1 small onion, chopped
- ½ celery rib, chopped
- 3 tablespoons cornstarch or arrowroot powder
- ½ cup water
- 1 tablespoon fresh sage, chopped
- 2 ½ pounds turkey breast, bone-in, skin on, trimmed of fat
- Salt to taste
- Black pepper powder to taste

Instructions:

1. Place a skillet over medium high heat. Add butter and allow it to melt. Add onion, celery, carrot and garlic and sauté for a few minutes until onion is translucent.
2. Add cornstarch and sauté for about a minute.
3. Add ½ cup broth and stir. Scrape the bottom of the pan to remove any browned bits that are stuck. Stir until the mixture is free from lumps. Turn off the heat.
4. Add remaining broth, wine, water, sage and bay leaves and stir. Transfer into the slow cooker.

5. Sprinkle salt and pepper all over the turkey and place in the slow cooker, with the skin side facing up.
6. Cover the pot and cook on low for 5-7 hours or on high for 2 ½ -3 ½ hours. The internal temperature of the turkey should show 165 degrees F (use an instant read thermometer at the thickest part of the meat)
7. Switch off the cooker.
8. Remove turkey and place on your cutting board. Cover the turkey loosely with foil.
9. Let the meat and the cooked liquids in the pot rest for 15 minutes.
10. Carefully discard the fat floating on the surface of the cooked liquid and strain into a saucepan. Discard the solids in the strainer.
11. Place saucepan over medium heat. Simmer until the gravy is thick.
12. Add salt and pepper to taste.
13. Remove the skin from the turkey and slice the turkey.
14. Serve turkey with gravy.

Arianna Brooks

Crockpot Turkey Breast

Makes: 3 servings

Carbs per serving: 3.7 grams (1 cup)

Ingredients:

- 1 bone-in turkey breast (2.5-3 pounds), skinless, thawed
- 1 yellow onion, chopped into chunks
- ½ cup chicken broth
- 3 tablespoons butter, divided, chilled, chopped into small cubes
- 3 stalks celery, chopped
- 6-8 baby carrots
- 2 teaspoons arrowroot powder or cornstarch mixed with a tablespoon water
- Cooking spray

For dry rub

- ½ tablespoon dried minced garlic
- ½ teaspoon paprika
- ½ teaspoon Italian seasoning
- A large pinch dried sage
- A large pinch dried parsley
- 1/8 teaspoon dried thyme
- ½ teaspoon seasoned salt
- ¼ teaspoon pepper powder

Instructions:

1. Grease the inside of the slow cooker by spraying with cooking spray.

2. Spread celery on the bottom of the cooker. Next place carrots. Drizzle chicken broth over it.
3. Mix together the dry rub mixture in a bowl. Rub this mixture over the turkey. Place the onion chunks and 2 tablespoons butter cubes inside the turkey at different places. Place turkey in the slow cooker, over the vegetables with the breast side facing down.
4. Melt remaining butter and brush it over the turkey.
5. Cover the pot and cook on Low for 5-7 hours or on High for 3 to 4 hours or until the internal temperature of the turkey shows 165 degree F (use an instant read thermometer at the thickest part of the meat)
6. Remove turkey with a slotted spoon and place on your cutting board. When cool enough to handle, remove the bone, slice and keep warm.
7. To make gravy: Let the liquid in the pot sit for a while. Carefully discard the fat that is floating on the top.
8. Uncover and cook on high for a while. Add arrowroot mixture and stir frequently until thick.
9. Taste and adjust the seasonings if required.
10. Serve turkey slices with gravy.

Arianna Brooks

Chapter Seven - Soups

Green Eggs & Ham Soup

Makes: 8 servings

Carbs per serving: 14 grams

Ingredients:

- 4 tablespoons extra-virgin olive oil, divided
- 1 large onion, chopped
- 8 cups low sodium chicken broth
- 4 cups cauliflower, chopped
- 8 cups baby spinach
- 6-7 cups water
- 8 large eggs
- 8 ounces thick cut ham or prosciutto, chopped
- 4 cloves garlic, minced
- 8 cups broccoli florets, chopped
- A handful fresh thyme leaves
- ½ cup fresh parsley, chopped + extra to garnish
- Salt to taste
- 5 teaspoons white vinegar

Instructions:

1. Place a skillet over medium heat. Add 2 tablespoons oil. When oil is heated, add ham and cook until light brown. Remove the meat and set aside on a plate.
2. Add 2 tablespoons oil. When the oil is heated, add onions and sauté until translucent.

3. Add garlic and sauté for few seconds until fragrant. Turn off the heat and transfer into the slow cooker.
4. Add broccoli, thyme, cauliflower, broth and salt into the cooker and stir.
5. Cover the pot and cook on Low for 2 hours or on High for 1 hour or until vegetables are very soft.
6. Add spinach and parsley and cook on Low for 1 hour or on High for 30 minutes or until the greens wilt.
7. Switch off the cooker and blend the contents of the pot with an immersion blender until smooth. Cover and keep warm.
8. Add water into a large saucepan. Add vinegar and place the saucepan over medium heat. When the water begins to just simmer. Take a spoon and simply swirl the water around.
9. Crack an egg into a bowl. Carefully slide the egg into the simmering water. Repeat this process with the remaining eggs. Poach the eggs in batches if required. Cook the eggs as per your liking.
10. Ladle soup into bowls. Divide ham pieces into the bowls. Remove the eggs with a slotted spoon and place in the soup bowl.
11. Garnish with parsley and serve.

Chicken-Corn Tortilla Soup

Makes: 4 servings

Carbs per serving: 14 grams

Ingredients:

- 1 cup onion, chopped
- ½ red bell pepper, deseeded, chopped
- 1 pound chicken thighs, bone-in, skinless
- 1 ½ cups water
- 1 teaspoon ground cumin
- ¼ teaspoon ground coriander
- 1 bay leaf
- ¼ cup corn, fresh or frozen, thaw if frozen
- 1 tablespoon lime juice
- 1 Anaheim or jalapeño pepper, deseeded, chopped
- 1 clove garlic, minced
- 2 cups low sodium chicken broth
- 7.5 oz. canned fire roasted diced tomatoes
- ¾ teaspoon dried oregano, crushed
- Salt to taste
- ½ cup tortilla chips, lightly crushed + extra for garnishing
- 1 teaspoon lime zest, grated

To serve

- Sour cream to drizzle
- ½ cup chopped avocado
- Lime wedges
- ½ cup Cheddar cheese, shredded

Instructions:

1. Add onion, red bell pepper, Anaheim pepper and garlic into the slow cooker.
2. Place chicken over it.
3. Pour broth and water. Add cumin, coriander, tomatoes, oregano, bay leaf and salt into the cooker. Stir until well combined.
4. Cover the pot and cook on low for 7 to 8 hours or on high for 3 ½ hours.
5. Remove chicken with a slotted spoon. Place on your cutting board. When cool enough to handle, shred the chicken with a pair of forks. Set aside.
6. Add tortilla chips and corn into the pot and stir. Cover and cook on high for 30 minutes.
7. Mix well so that the tortilla chips are broken.
8. Add shredded chicken, lime juice and lime zest and mix well.
9. Ladle into soup bowls. Sprinkle avocado and cheese. Drizzle sour cream and serve with lime wedges.

Rainbow Vegetable Soup

Makes: 6 servings

Carbs per serving: 10 grams

Ingredients:

- 1 medium turnip, peeled, diced
- 1 small carrot, diced (optional)
- ½ pound green beans, fresh or frozen
- 7.5 oz. pumpkin puree
- ½ pound spinach, fresh or frozen
- ½ small onion, chopped
- ½ cup celery leaves, chopped
- 3 celery stalks, chopped
- 1 cup water
- A pinch rubbed sage
- A large pinch chopped thyme
- 4 cups vegetable broth
- Salt to taste

Instructions:

1. Add turnip, carrot, beans, pumpkin puree, onion, celery, water, sage, thyme and salt into the slow cooker.
2. Cover the pot and cook on Low for 4 hours or on High for 2 hours.
3. Add spinach and stir. Cover and let it rest for 5-6 minutes.
4. Ladle into soup bowls and serve.

Arianna Brooks

Slow-Cooker Hot & Sour Soup

Makes: 3 servings

Carbs per serving: 11 grams

Ingredients:

- 1 can (14.5 ounces) chicken broth
- ½ can (from an 8 ounce can) bamboo shoots, drained
- ¼ cup water
- 1 ½ tablespoons rice vinegar or white vinegar
- ½ teaspoon brown sugar
- 1 tablespoon cornstarch mixed with a tablespoon cold water
- 2 ounces refrigerated water packed firm tofu, drained, cut into cubes
- 1 medium carrot, sliced on the bias
- ½ can (from an 8 ounce can) water chestnuts, drained
- 2 oz. mushrooms, sliced
- ½ tablespoon soy sauce
- Crushed red pepper to taste
- 4 oz. frozen peeled and deveined shrimp, uncooked
- 1 tablespoon chopped parsley or cilantro

Instructions:

1. Add broth, bamboo shoots, water, rice vinegar, brown sugar, carrot, water chestnuts, mushroom, soy sauce and crushed red pepper into the slow cooker.
2. Cover the pot and cook on low for 6-8 hours or on high for 3 to 4 hours.
3. Add cornstarch mixture and stir. Stir in the shrimp and tofu.

4. Cover the pot and cook on high for 30 minutes.
5. Ladle into soup bowls and serve.

Arianna Brooks

Barbecue Meatball Soup

Makes: 3 servings

Carbs per serving: 14 grams

Ingredients:

- ½ pound 90% lean ground beef
- 2 tablespoons refrigerated or frozen egg product, thawed
- Black pepper powder to taste
- 1 medium carrot, thinly sliced
- 1 medium bell pepper of any color, cut into thin strips
- 2 cloves garlic, minced
- 2 tablespoons smoked paprika or sweet paprika
- 1 stalk celery, thinly sliced
- 1 small onion, chopped
- 1 ½ cups water
- ¼ cup light barbecue sauce
- ¼ cup crumbled reduced fat blue cheese
- ½ tablespoon canola oil
- ½ cup beef broth
- 6 tablespoons soft whole wheat bread crumbs
- 1 ½ cups collard greens, trimmed, chopped (or use mustard greens or kale)
- Cooking spray

Instructions:

1. To make meatballs: Add breadcrumbs, beef, garlic, egg, paprika and pepper into a bowl and stir until well combined. Make 12 portions of the mixture and shape each into balls.

Slow Cooker Low Carb

2. Grease the bottom of the slow cooker by spraying with cooking spray. Place meatballs in it.
3. Cover the pot and cook on high for 1 hour.
4. Meanwhile, place a pan over medium heat. Add oil. When the oil is heated, add onion, celery, carrot and bell pepper and sauté for 2-3 minutes.
5. Turn off the heat. Stir in the broth, barbecue sauce and water and transfer into the slow cooker.
6. Cover the pot and cook on high for 30 minutes. Add collard greens during the last 5 minutes of cooking.
7. Ladle into soup bowls. Place 4 meatballs in each bowl. Garnish with blue cheese and serve.

Arianna Brooks

Inestrone Soup with Pork

Makes: 6 servings

Carbs per serving: 10 grams

Ingredients:

- 1 tablespoon avocado oil or olive oil
- 1 medium carrot, peeled, diced
- 1 zucchini, diced
- 2 cloves garlic, minced
- 1 medium sweet potato, peeled, cubed
- 1 stalk celery, chopped
- 2 shallots, diced
- 1 cup frozen spinach or 2 cups packed fresh spinach, chopped
- ¾ pound ground pork, crumbled
- 1 can (14.5 ounces) diced tomatoes
- 2 cups low sodium vegetable stock
- 1 cup water
- 1 bay leaf
- ½ teaspoon dried basil
- 1 teaspoon dried oregano
- ½ teaspoon dried parsley
- Sea salt to taste
- ¼ teaspoon cayenne pepper or to taste

Instructions:

1. Place a skillet over medium heat. Add oil. When the oil is heated, add shallot and garlic and sauté until translucent. Transfer into the slow cooker.

2. Add carrot, zucchini, sweet potato, celery, pork, tomatoes, garlic, stock, water, bay leaf, herbs, salt and cayenne pepper. Stir until well combined.
3. Cover the pot and cook on low for 6 to 7 hours or on high for 3 – 3 ½ hours.
4. Add spinach. Mix well. Cover and let it sit for a few minutes until spinach wilts. Discard the bay leaves.
5. Ladle into soup bowls and serve.

Arianna Brooks

Curried Butternut Squash Soup

Makes: 4 servings

Carbs per serving: 15 grams

Ingredients:

- 1 ¼ pounds butternut squash, peeled, deseeded, chopped
- 1 small onion, chopped
- 2 cloves garlic, chopped or ½ teaspoon garlic powder
- 7 oz. coconut milk
- Fresh cilantro, chopped to garnish
- 1 ½ cups vegetable stock or chicken stock
- 2 teaspoons curry powder
- Sea salt to taste
- Pepper powder to taste
- Lime juice to taste

Instructions:

1. Add squash, onion, garlic, stock, curry powder, salt and pepper into the slow cooker and stir.
2. Cover the pot and cook on low for 6 to 7 hours or on high for 3 to 3 ½ hours.
3. Add coconut milk. Mix well. Using a stick blender, blend until smooth. Add lime juice and stir.
4. Ladle into soup bowls.
5. Garnish with cilantro and serve.

Asparagus & Sorrel Bisque

Makes: 4 servings

Carbs per serving: 9 grams

Ingredients:

- 1 tablespoons unsalted butter
- 1 large leek, thinly sliced, white and pale green only
- ½ teaspoon kosher salt
- Pepper powder to taste
- 1 pound asparagus, trimmed, cut into ½ inch pieces
- ¼ cup crème fraiche
- 1 tablespoon extra-virgin olive oil
- 1 stalk green garlic, sliced
- 2 cups low sodium vegetable or no chicken broth
- 2 cups sorrel or baby arugula + extra to garnish
- 1 radish, sliced, to garnish

Instructions:

1. Add oil and butter into a small pan. Place pan over medium heat. Turn off the heat when the butter melts.
2. Transfer into the slow cooker.
3. Add leeks, green garlic, asparagus, salt, pepper and broth.
4. Cover the pot and cook on low for 2-3 hours or on high for 1 to 1 ½ hours or until asparagus is tender.
5. Switch off the slow cooker and cool completely.
6. Pour soup into a bowl and place in the refrigerator for 2 hours. Do not cover the bowl during this time.
7. Remove the bowl from the refrigerator and transfer the soup into a blender.

8. Add sorrel and blend for 40 to 50 seconds or until smooth.
9. Taste and adjust the seasoning if required.
10. Ladle into soup bowls. Sprinkle some pepper on top.
11. Place radish slices on top and serve.

Slow Cooker Low Carb

Creamy Chicken Noodle Soup

Makes: 8 servings

Carbs per serving: 12 grams

Ingredients:

- 2 1/2 cups chicken, chopped & cooked (about 12 ounces)
- 32 fluid ounces reduced-sodium chicken broth (1 container)
- 2 cups dried egg noodles
- 1 1/2 cups fresh mushrooms, sliced (4 ounces)
- 1/4 cup onion (chopped)
- 1 1/2 cups sliced carrots (3 medium carrots should do)
- 3/4 teaspoon garlic-pepper seasoning
- 1 1/2 cups sliced celery stalks (3 stalks should do)
- 3 ounces reduced-fat cream Neufchâtel cheese (cut up)
- 1 1/2 teaspoons crushed dried thyme
- 3 cups water

Instructions:

1. Pour the chicken broth into the slow cooker and add water to it.
2. Add the chicken, mushrooms, onions, carrots, garlic-pepper seasoning, celery and thyme to the broth-water mixture in the cooker
3. Cook on high for 4 hours or low heat for 8 hours.
4. In case you are cooking on low, increase to high setting after 8 hours and add the cream cheese.
5. Stir well until combined and add the uncooked egg noodles to the cooker.

6. Cover and cook for 30 minutes until the noodles become tender.
7. If you have been cooking on high, just add the cream cheese and follow step 5 and step 6
8. Turn off heat and mix the contents thoroughly before you transfer to a bowl.
9. Serve warm and enjoy!

Slow Cooker Low Carb

Ginger-Chicken Noodle Soup

Makes: 6 servings

Carbs per serving: 13 grams

Ingredients:

- 1/2 teaspoon ground ginger or 1 teaspoon grated fresh ginger
- 1 pound chicken thighs (skinless, boneless), cut into 1-inch pieces
- 2 ounces dried medium noodles or rice vermicelli noodles
- 6 ounces pea pods (frozen), thawed and halved diagonally
- 2 coarsely shredded medium carrots
- 14 ounces chicken broth (3 cans)
- 2 tablespoons dry sherry
- 1 tablespoon soy sauce + extra for serving
- 1/4 teaspoon black pepper (ground)
- 1 tablespoon rice vinegar
- 1 cup water

Instructions:

1. Pour the chicken broth into the slow cooker and add one cup of water to it.
2. Add the chicken, carrots, sherry, soy sauce, pepper, ginger and rice vinegar to the broth-water mixture in the cooker
3. Stir well until combined. Cover the cooker and cook on high for 3 hours.

4. Once the cooking cycle is over, add the pea pods and noodles to the contents in the cooker. Stir once.
5. Cover the cooker and cook on high for 10 minutes until the noodles become tender.
6. Ladle the soup into a bowl and serve hot with soy sauce. Enjoy!

Roasted Tomato and Vegetable Soup

Makes: 8 servings

Carbs per serving: 15 grams

Ingredients:

- 1-cup cauliflower florets and/or small broccoli (you can use 1 cup cauliflower or 1 cup broccoli or 1 cup of mixed cauliflower-broccoli.)
- 14.5 ounces fire-roasted diced tomatoes (1 can)
- 19 ounces rinsed and drained cannellini beans (1 can)
- 1 medium carrot (chopped)
- 1 medium onion (chopped)
- 1 small zucchini (cut lengthwise and slice)
- 1 celery stalk, sliced
- 2 cups butternut squash (cubed and peeled)
- 43.5 ounces reduced-sodium chicken broth (3 cans)
- 2 teaspoons crushed dried oregano
- 1 teaspoon minced garlic (2 bottled garlic cloves)
- 1/4 teaspoon black pepper (freshly ground)
- 1 tablespoon olive oil
- Freshly shredded Parmesan cheese (for garnishing)
- 1/4 teaspoon salt

Instructions:

1. Add oil to the slow cooker and combine the garlic, dried oregano, squash, celery, carrot, onion, beans, tomatoes and chicken broth in it.
2. Cover the cooker and cook on high for 4 hours and low for 8 hours.

3. Once the cooking cycle is over, add the broccoli or cauliflower, zucchini, pepper and salt. Mix well.
4. Cover and cook for additional 30 minutes on the high heat setting.
5. Transfer the soup into a bowl and sprinkle the shredded Parmesan cheese.
6. Serve hot and enjoy!

Low-Carb Pumpkin and Coconut Soup

Makes: 6 servings

Carbs per serving: 11.4 grams

Ingredients:

- 17 ounces pumpkin chunks
- 1 1/2 coconut cream + extra for garnishing
- 1 diced medium onion
- 4 tablespoons butter
- 1 teaspoon crushed ginger
- 2 cups vegetable stock
- 1 teaspoon crushed garlic
- Salt and pepper, to taste

Instructions:

1. Grease the insides of the slow cooker with 1 tablespoon melted butter.
2. Add the pumpkin chunks, onion, ginger and garlic into the cooker.
3. Add the coconut cream, remaining butter and vegetable stock to the contents in the cooker.
4. Sprinkle with salt and pepper. Mix well until the contents are thoroughly combined.
5. Cover the cooker and cook on high heat for 6 hours or on low heat setting for 8 hours
6. Once the cooking cycle is over, puree the mixture carefully with an immersion blender.
7. Transfer to a large bowl. Ladle the soup to the serving bowl and garnish with coconut cream.
8. Serve warm and enjoy!

Arianna Brooks

Pumpkin Soup

Makes: 3 servings

Carbs per serving: 13 grams

Ingredients:

- 1/8 cup finely chopped green bell pepper
- 1/4 cup finely chopped onion
- 1/2 cup low sodium vegetable broth
- 1 cup pureed pumpkin
- 1 cup skim milk
- 1/8 tsp thyme
- 1/8 tsp nutmeg

Instructions:

1. Mix all of the ingredients together in the slow cooker.
2. Cover and cook for 5 hours on low.

Tomato Soup

Makes: 3 servings

Carbs per serving: 9 grams

Ingredients:

- 2 1/2 cups diced tomatoes
- 1/2 Tbsp. unsalted tomato paste
- 2 cups low sodium vegetable broth
- 1/4 cup minced onion
- 1/2 Tbsp. minced garlic
- 1/2 tsp basil
- 1/8 tsp black pepper

Instructions:

1. Mix together all of the ingredients in the slow cooker.
2. Cover and cook for 6 hours on low, stirring once.

Arianna Brooks

Cauliflower Soup

Makes: 3 servings

Carbs per serving: 10 grams

Ingredients:

- 2 cup diced cauliflower
- 4 oz. fat free cream cheese
- 1 cup water
- 1/4 cup shredded cheddar
- 1/4 cup potato flakes

Instructions:

1. Pour the water into a saucepan and place the cauliflower in it. Place over medium high heat and bring to a boil. Turn off the heat.
2. Place the cream and cheddar cheeses inside the slow cooker, then add the cauliflower and boiled water. Stir well.
3. Add the potato flakes and stir to combined, then cover and cook for 2 hours on low.

Broccoli Soup

Makes: 2 to 3 servings

Carbs per serving: 15 grams

Ingredients:

- 1 lb. broccoli, chopped
- 1 1/2 cups water
- 1/2 cup skim milk
- 1/4 cup cheddar cheese, sliced into cubes

Instructions:

1. Combine the chopped broccoli and water in the slow cooker. Cover and cook for 1 hour on high.
2. Stir in the skim milk and cook for extra 10 minutes. Add the cheese and stir until the cheese melts.

Arianna Brooks

Mexican Chicken Chowder

Makes: 4 servings

Carbs per serving: 10.3 grams

Ingredients:

- ½ can cream of chicken soup
- ½ can yellow corn
- ½ pound boneless, skinless chicken breasts, chopped into small pieces
- ¾ can jalapeno and cheddar cheese dip
- ½ can fat free chicken broth
- ¼ cup canned green chilies
- ½ cup light sour cream

Instructions:

1. Add corn, chicken soup, chicken broth and green chilies without juice into the slow cooker.
2. Add chicken pieces and mix well.
3. Cover and cook on low for 4 hours
4. In a bowl mix together sour cream, cheese dip and 1 cup of the soup from the cooker. Mix well and pour it back to the cooker.
5. Cook on low for 15 minutes more.
6. Ladle into soup bowls and serve hot.

Summer Vegetable Soup

Makes: 4 servings

Carbs per serving: 14 grams

Ingredients:

- 2 cups low sodium vegetable broth
- 4 oz. frozen corn
- 4 oz. frozen green beans
- 1/4 cup chopped carrots
- 1/2 cup sliced zucchini
- 1 cup chopped tomatoes
- 1/4 cup chopped onions
- 1/4 tsp thyme
- 1/4 tsp minced garlic
- 1/4 tsp basil
- 1/8 tsp black pepper
- 1/2 cup chopped broccoli
- 1/4 cup frozen peas

Instructions:

1. Mix together all of the ingredients, except the frozen peas and broccoli, in the slow cooker.
2. Cover and cook for 3 hours on high, or for 6 hours on low.
3. Add the broccoli and cook for an extra 30 minutes on high. Add the peas and cook for an extra 10 minutes on high.

Arianna Brooks

California-Style Seafood Soup

Makes: 3 servings

Carbs per serving: 10 grams

Ingredients:

- 7 1/2 oz. undrained diced tomatoes
- 1/2 cup water
- 1/2 cup clam juice
- 1/4 cup dry white wine or clam juice
- 1/2 cup thinly sliced onion
- 1/2 cup thinly sliced green onion
- 1/2 cup thinly sliced green bell pepper
- 1/2 Tbsp. olive oil
- 1/2 Tbsp. minced garlic
- 1/4 tsp dried tarragon
- 1/4 tsp rosemary
- 1/4 tsp thyme
- 1/2 bay leaf
- 1/2 lb. crab meat or firm white fish, cubed
- 6 oz. shrimp, peeled and deveined
- 10 clams in shells, scrubbed
- 1/8 tsp salt
- 1/4 tsp black pepper

Instructions:

1. In the slow cooker, mix together all of the ingredients, except the seafood, salt, and pepper.
2. Cover and cook for 6 hours on low. Add the seafood within the last 15 minutes of cooking time.

3. Remove the bay leaf and unopened clams. Stir in the salt and pepper.

Arianna Brooks

Spicy Chicken Soup

Makes: 8 servings

Carbs per serving: 9.7 grams

Ingredients:

- 4 cups of water
- ½ of a large onion, chopped
- 3 chicken breasts
- ¼ of a large cabbage, shredded
- 1 can of diced green chilies, undrained
- 1 can of stewed tomatoes, undrained
- 1 cup of salsa
- 4 tbsp. of heavy whipping cream
- 18 oz. of cream cheese, softened
- 1 tbsp. of garlic salt
- 1 tbsp. of ground cumin
- Salt
- Pepper

Instructions:

1. Add the chicken breasts, cabbage, onion and water into the slow cooker.
2. Cook for 4 hours over high settings or 8 hours on low. Once done, remove the chicken from the slow cooker and shred into smaller pieces.
3. Replace the chicken into the slow cooker and add in the green chilies, tomatoes, salsa, whipping cream, cream cheese, garlic salt, ground cumin, pepper and salt.
4. Mix well and cook until the cream cheese completely incorporates into the soup.

Moqueca de Camaroes (Brazilian Shrimp Soup)

Makes: 3 servings

Carbs per serving: 5 grams

Ingredients:

- ¾ pound raw shrimp, peeled, deveined
- 2 tablespoons olive oil
- 2 tablespoons onions, diced
- 1 clove garlic, minced
- 2 tablespoons roasted red peppers, diced
- 2 tablespoons fresh cilantro, chopped
- 7 ounce can diced tomatoes
- ½ cup coconut milk
- 2 ½ cups water
- 1 tablespoon Sriracha chilli sauce
- 1 tablespoon fresh lime juice
- Salt to taste
- Pepper to taste

Ingredients:

1. Place a skillet over medium heat. Add olive oil. When oil is heated, add onions and sauté until translucent. Add garlic and pepper. Sauté for a minute and transfer to the slow cooker.
2. Add tomatoes, shrimps, cilantro, and water.
3. Cover and cook on low for 3-4 hours.
4. Add coconut milk, Sriracha sauce, salt, and pepper. Cook on low for 10 more minutes.
5. Serve immediately garnished with cilantro.

Arianna Brooks

Pizza Soup

Makes: 4 servings

Carbs per serving: 12.7 grams

Ingredients:

- 8 ounce canned crushed tomatoes
- 1 can (16 ounce) beef broth
- 1 can (16 ounce) mushrooms
- 1 small green pepper, diced
- 1 small onion, diced
- ½ pound Italian sausage
- ¼ pound pepperoni, thinly sliced
- ½ teaspoon garlic powder
- 1 teaspoon dried oregano
- 1 teaspoon Italian seasoning
- ½ cup mozzarella cheese, grated
- 2 tablespoons parmesan, grated

Instructions:

1. Place a nonstick skillet over medium heat. Add the sausage and cook until browned.
2. Remove the sausage with a slotted spoon and add to the slow cooker.
3. Add rest of the ingredients except cheeses to the cooker.
4. Cover and cook on low for 6-8 hours.
5. Ladle into soup bowls. Garnish with cheese and serve hot.

Slow Cooker Low Carb

Cheese Burger Soup

Makes: 4 servings

Carbs per serving: 14.67 grams

Ingredients:

- 1 pound ground beef
- 2 ¼ cups beef broth
- 12 ounce tomato paste
- 2 tomatoes, chopped
- 1 red bell pepper, chopped
- 2 sticks celery, chopped
- ¾ cup onions, chopped
- 2 teaspoons parsley
- 1 ½ teaspoon Worcestershire sauce
- 1 ½ teaspoon garlic powder
- ¾ teaspoon salt or to taste
- ¾ teaspoon pepper powder
- ¾ cup cheese, grated
- 3 slices bacon, cooked, chopped

Instructions:

1. Place a nonstick skillet over medium heat. Add the beef and cook until browned.
2. When beef is lightly browned, remove as much fat as possible.
3. Add onions, pepper, and celery. Sauté for 2-3 minutes and transfer the contents to the slow cooker.
4. Add rest of the ingredients, mix well. If you want your soup thinner, then add some more beef broth or water.

5. Cover and cook on low for 6-8 hours. Stir in between if possible.
6. Ladle soup into bowls. Add bacon and top with cheese.

Slow Cooker Low Carb

Spicy Thai Chicken Soup

Makes: 4 servings

Carbs per serving: 9 grams

Ingredients:

- 1 teaspoon vegetable canola oil
- 2 cups mushrooms, sliced
- 1 cup carrots, diagonally sliced
- 1 medium onion, chopped
- ½ medium red bell pepper, chopped into thin strips
- 2 tablespoons fresh ginger, peeled, minced
- 5 cloves garlic, minced
- 6 inch piece of lemongrass, halved lengthwise
- 1 tablespoon red curry paste or more if you like it spicier
- 3 cups chicken stock or low sodium chicken broth
- 1 cup coconut thin milk
- 1 tablespoon fish sauce
- 1 tablespoon sugar (optional)
- 4 cups boneless, skinless chicken breast or thighs
- 1 cup green onions, cut into thin strips
- ¼ cup fresh basil, chopped
- 2 tablespoons fresh lime juice
- Cooking spray

Instructions:

1. Place a nonstick skillet over medium heat. Add oil and heat. Add the chicken and cook until brown on both the sides.

2. Spray the slow cooker with cooking spray. Add onions, carrots, bell pepper, garlic, ginger, fish sauce and curry paste. Mix well.
3. Place the browned chicken over the vegetables. Add broth all over the chicken.
4. Cover and set the cooker on low for 5 hours or until done.
5. Using a slotted spoon, remove the chicken and shred it using forks.
6. Add the shredded chicken back to the pot. Add rest of the ingredients except lime juice. Cook on low for another 30 minutes or until the mushrooms are cooked.
7. Add lime juice. Mix well and serve immediately.

Turkey Soup

Makes: 6 servings

Carbs per serving: 4.8 grams

Ingredients:

Broth:
- 1 turkey breast
- 1 small onion, chopped
- 1 stick celery, chopped
- 1 small carrot, chopped
- ¼ teaspoon salt or to taste
- ¼ teaspoon pepper powder
- 1 bay leaf
- ½ teaspoon poultry seasoning
- 1 teaspoon instant chicken bouillon granules
- 6 cups water

Soup:
- 1 onion, chopped
- 2 cloves garlic, minced
- 1 carrot, peeled, chopped
- 1 stalk celery, chopped
- ½ teaspoon dried thyme
- ¼ teaspoon salt
- 1 tablespoon fresh parsley leaves
- 1 cup shredded turkey

Instructions:

1. To make the broth: Add all the ingredients of the broth to the slow cooker and cook on low for 8 hours.
2. Strain the broth and pour the liquid back to the cooker. Shred the cooked turkey and add it back to the cooker.
3. Add rest of the ingredients except parsley.
4. Cover and cook on high for 3 ½ hours. Add parsley and cook for 30 minutes more.
5. Ladle soup into bowls and serve immediately.

Onion Soup

Makes: 8 servings

Carbs per serving: 7.4 grams

Ingredients:

- 4 sweet onions, sliced
- 1 tbsp. of Worcestershire sauce
- 2 tbsp. of butter
- 1 tbsp. of balsamic vinegar
- 2 tsp of brown sugar
- 3 cloves of garlic, minced
- ½ tsp of pepper
- 3 tbsp. of all-purpose flour
- ½ tsp of salt
- 64 oz. of beef broth
- 2 tbsp. of fresh thyme

Instructions:

1. Turn on the slow cooker and set it on high. Add in the butter, onions, vinegar, Worcestershire sauce, brown sugar, pepper, garlic and salt. Cook for 1 hour while stirring occasionally.
2. Once done, add in the flour and cook for another five minutes.
3. Then, add in the thyme and beef broth and cover. Cook for 8 hours on high setting.

Arianna Brooks

Chicken Fajita Soup

Makes: 14 servings

Carbs per serving: 4 grams

Ingredients:

- 1 ½ lbs. of chicken breast
- 14.5 oz. of diced tomatoes
- 32 oz. of chicken stock
- 1 medium yellow bell pepper, diced
- 1 medium onion, diced
- 1 medium orange bell pepper, diced
- 6 oz. of mushrooms, sliced thinly
- 4 tbsp. of taco seasoning
- 4 cloves of garlic, minced
- 2 tbsp. of fresh cilantro, chopped
- 1 tbsp. garlic salt

Instructions:

1. Place the chicken breast, chicken stock, diced tomatoes, yellow bell pepper, orange bell pepper, onion, mushrooms, garlic, taco seasoning, cilantro and garlic salt inside the slow cooker.
2. Cover and cook for 6 hours on low setting. Once done, shred the chicken meat using a fork and give it a quick stir. Replace the cover and cook for another hour.

Slow Cooker Low Carb

Italian Sausage and Lentil Soup

Makes: 16 servings

Carbs per serving: 4.9 grams

Ingredients:

- Salt and pepper
- 2 tbsp. of red wine vinegar
- 2 tbsp. of Dijon mustard
- ½ cup of parmesan, grated
- 1 cup of heavy cream
- 1 rib of celery, diced
- 1 leek, cleaned then trimmed
- 3 tbsp. of garlic, minced
- ½ cup of onion, diced
- ½ cup of carrot, diced
- 1 cup of spinach
- 1 ½ cups of lentils
- 5 cups of chicken stock
- 2 tbsp. of olive oil
- 2 tbsp. of butter
- 1 ½lb of Italian sausage

Instructions:

1. Set the slow cooker on low heat and turn it on. Rinse the lentils thoroughly and add it into the slow cooker together with the chicken stock.
2. In a skillet placed on medium-high heat, add in the butter and olive oil and cook the sausage until it's browned. Remove the sausage from the skillet using a slotted spoon and reserve the cooking liquid. Add the cooked sausage into the slow cooker.

3. Add in the celery, leek, garlic, onions, carrots, and spinach into the skillet and season everything using the pepper and salt. Cook the vegetables for 10 minutes and add it into the slow cooker and stir.
4. Stir in the red wine vinegar, Dijon mustard, Parmesan cheese, and heavy cream into the slow cooker. Cover and cook for 8 hours on low settings.

Rueben Soup

Makes: 14 servings

Carbs per serving: 4 grams

Ingredients:

- 1 ½ cups of Swiss cheese, shredded
- 2 cups of heavy cream
- ¾ tsp. of black pepper
- 1 tsp. of caraway seeds
- 1 tsp. of sea salt
- 1 cup of sauerkraut
- 32oz of beef stock
- 1lb of corned beef, chopped
- 3 tbsp. of butter
- 2 cloves of garlic (large), minced
- 2 ribs of celery, diced
- 1 onion (medium), diced

Instructions:

1. Preheat the slow cooker and set it on high setting.
2. In a pan, add in the butter, garlic, celery, and onion and cook on low-medium heat. Once the onion becomes translucent and soft, transfer the contents of the pan into the slow cooker.
3. Add in the black pepper, caraway seeds, sea salt, sauerkraut, beef stock, and corned beef to the slow cooker. Cover and cook for 4 ½ hours on high settings.
4. Once done, stir in the Swiss cheese and heavy cream and cook for another hour.

Arianna Brooks

Mulligatawny Soup

Makes: 4 servings

Carbs per serving: 15 grams

Ingredients:

- ½ a medium tart apple, peeled, chopped
- 1 small carrot, chopped
- 1 stalk celery, chopped
- 1 small onion, chopped
- 2 tablespoons butter, chopped
- 2 ½ tablespoons all-purpose flour
- ¼ cup water
- 1 teaspoon curry powder
- ¼ teaspoon sugar
- ¼ teaspoon salt or to taste
- 1/8 teaspoon pepper
- 1/8 teaspoon ground mace
- 3 cups chicken broth
- ½ cup cooked chicken, chopped
- 1 small tomato, peeled, seeded, chopped
- 1 small green bell pepper, chopped
- 2 whole cloves
- ½ tablespoon fresh parsley, chopped
- ½ cup cooked rice

Instructions:

1. Add all the ingredients except rice, flour, and water to the slow cooker.
2. Cover and cook on low for about 5 hours. (If you are using uncooked chicken, then cook for 7-8 hours)

3. Mix water and flour and add to the cooker, stirring constantly. Add rice and cook for another 30 minutes on low.
4. Discard the cloves and serve hot in soup bowls.

Arianna Brooks

Spinach, Tomato, Vegetable Soup

Makes: 5 servings

Carbs per serving: 7.2 grams

Ingredients:

- 5 ounce baby spinach
- 1 medium carrot, chopped
- 1 medium celery stalk, chopped
- 1 medium onion, chopped
- 1 clove garlic, minced
- 2 cups vegetable broth
- 14 ounce canned, diced tomatoes
- 1 bay leaf
- ½ tablespoon dried basil
- ½ teaspoon dried oregano
- ¼ teaspoon red pepper flakes, crushed

Instructions:

1. Add all the ingredients to the slow cooker. Mix well.
2. Cover and cook on low for 7-8 hours or high for 3-4 hours.
3. Serve hot in soup bowls.

Vegetable Soup

Makes: 8 servings

Carbs per serving: 13.1 grams

Ingredients:

- 1 medium zucchini, cubed
- 4 cloves garlic, chopped
- 2 stalks celery, chopped
- 1 cup frozen broccoli
- 3 medium carrots, sliced
- 1 small parsnip, sliced
- Salt to taste
- Red pepper flakes to taste
- ¼ cup tomato paste
- 5 cups water
- ½ tablespoon olive oil

Instructions:

1. Add olive oil to the slow cooker. Add onions and sauté until it turns translucent.
2. Add rest of the ingredients.
3. Cover and cook on low for 4 hours.
4. Serve hot.

Arianna Brooks

Zucchini Soup

Makes: 4 servings

Carbs per serving: 4.3 grams

Ingredients:

- 3 medium-sized green zucchini squash, chopped w/ peel
- 2 cups beef or chicken broth
- 1 tbsp. butter
- 1/2 cup yellow onion, chopped
- 1/2 tsp salt
- 1/4 tsp pepper
- 1 tbsp. regular whipping cream

Instructions:

1. Combine all ingredients in the slow cooker, except for the whipping cream.
2. Allow to cook over low heat for about 5 hours or until the zucchini is tender and soft.
3. Using a blender (preferably a stick blender you can use in the crockpot), puree the soup completely.
4. Stir the whipping cream in.
5. Immediately serve and enjoy!

Minestrone Veggie Soup

Makes: 8 to 10 servings

Carbs per serving: 4.15 grams

Ingredients:

- 2 cloves of garlic, chopped
- 2 cups celery, chopped
- 1 medium yellow onion, chopped
- 1 cup broccoli, chopped
- 1/4 cup fresh parsley, chopped
- 2 cups zucchini squash, quartered and chopped
- 2 cups cauliflower (frozen or fresh), chopped
- 3 cubes beef bouillon
- 1 small handful basil and sage, fresh and finely chopped
- 5 cups water (just a bit more than enough to cover the vegetables)
- 3/4 cup parmesan cheese, grated
- Salt & pepper to taste

Instructions:

1. Place all ingredients in the slow cooker, except for the Parmesan cheese.
2. Cook over slow heat setting for at least 8 hours or until the veggies are soft and tender.
3. Remove 2 cups of veggies and process with a food processor or immersion stick blender.
4. Put the vegetable puree back into the cooker to thicken and give texture to the soup without adding any carbs.
5. Turn off the crock-pot and allow the soup to slightly cool down.
6. Mix the Parmesan cheese into the soup.

7. Serve while soup is hot.

Cream of Asparagus Soup

Makes: 3 to 4 servings

Carbs per serving: 4 grams

Ingredients:

- 2 cups chicken broth
- 1 lb. asparagus, trimmed, washed and chopped into 3
- 1/2 cup yellow onion, chopped
- 1/2 tsp salt
- 1/4 tsp pepper
- 2 tbsp. butter

Instructions:

1. Combine all the ingredients in the slow cooker.
2. Allow to cook for about 4 hours over high heat setting or until the asparagus becomes very tender.
3. Puree the soup completely with a blender.

Arianna Brooks

Chicken Parmesan Soup

Makes: 4 serving

Carbs per serving: 3.9 grams

Ingredients:

- 2 skinless, boneless chicken breasts, diced
- 4 cups chicken stock or chicken broth
- 1/3 cup parmesan cheese, grated
- 1 cup water
- 1/8 tsp pepper
- 1/2 tsp seasoned or regular salt
- 1 cup zucchini, diced
- 1/8 cup of freshly chopped parsley
- 1 medium-sized yellow onion, chopped
- 2 stalks celery, diced
- 1 tsp bouillon beef base
- 1/4 tsp nutmeg

Instructions:

1. Set aside the Parmesan, chicken, and nutmeg. Place the rest of the ingredients in the slow cooker.
2. Cover the cooker and allow to cook for about 4 to 5 hours on low (3 hours on high heat setting).
3. Put the chicken and nutmeg in the cooker and cook for 1 hour more or until the chicken breasts are tender and cooked through.
4. Put the Parmesan cheese into the broth. Stir until the cheese melts and the soup absorbs the flavor.
5. Add salt & pepper as necessary.
6. Serve hot.

Italian Low Carb Wedding Soup

Makes: 6 servings

Carbs per serving: 1 gram

Ingredients:

For the Meatballs

- 1 small-sized yellow onion, grated and w/ extra juice squeezed out
- 1 egg
- 1/3 cup fresh Italian parsley, chopped
- 3/4 cup parmesan cheese, grated
- 1 tsp garlic powder
- 1/2 lb. ground beef and 1/2 lb. ground pork (1 lb. meatloaf mix)
- 1/2 tsp black pepper

For the Soup

- 12 cups chicken broth (low sodium)
- 2 eggs
- 1/2 tsp nutmeg
- 1 large-sized head of curly endive, chopped (in case endive is unavailable, substitute with kale, escarole or a few handfuls of spinach)
- 2 tbsp. parmesan cheese, grated

Instructions:

1. Wash the curly endive, chop (1" pcs), then set aside.
2. Create mini meatballs. To do it, mix all meatball ingredients in a bowl. With clean hands, roll the mini meatballs at around 1 tsp each. They will plump up a bit

when cooked; you should be able to make around 60 mini meatballs.
3. Prepare the soup. To do it, Boil the nutmeg and chicken broth in a large-sized pot. Put the uncooked mini meatballs in. Lower the heat down into a simmer, and allow to cook for about 4 minutes.
4. Stir the curly endive in, and simmer for 4 minutes more until the meatballs are done and cooked through.
5. Whisk together the eggs and Parmesan cheese in a small-sized bowl. Sprinkle the egg mixture slowly into the broth as you stir the broth. Stir in a figure 8 motion using a fork to form thin strands.
6. Remove from the heat and put salt & pepper, as necessary. Serve topped with some grated Parmesan cheese.

Hot Chicken Cabbage Soup

Makes: 20 serving

Carbs per serving: 5.5 grams

Ingredients:

- 1 medium-sized cabbage head, shredded
- 4 skinless, boneless chicken breasts, cut in cubes
- 1 cup of celery, sliced
- 1 large-sized onion, diced
- 10 cups of water
- 10 tsp chicken consommé, dry
- 2 cups chicken stock
- 2 tbsp. oregano
- 2 tbsp. basil
- 3 cloves garlic
- 4 tsp of hot pepper sauce, to taste

Instructions:

1. Make sure the ingredients are sliced, diced, or cubed to required size.
2. Put all the ingredients in the crockpot and cook for 8 to 10 hours on low heat setting.
3. Serve preferably with whole grain bread. Enjoy

Arianna Brooks

Split Pea & Ham Soup

Makes: 8 serving

Carbs per serving: 14.5 grams

Ingredients:

- 1 lb. dried split peas
- 1 cup celery, sliced
- 1 cup carrots, sliced
- 1 cup onions, sliced
- 2 cups cooked ham, sliced and diced
- 6 cups water
- 1 tbsp. seasoning (Nature's Seasons), to taste

Instructions:

1. Put all the ingredients in the slow cooker.
2. Place the cover and allow to cook for around 4 hours.
3. Serve hot.

Chapter Eight – Dips, Stews, Snacks & Sausages

Lamb Ropa Vieja (Cuban Lamb Stew)

Makes: 5 servings

Carbs per serving: 6 grams

Ingredients:

- 2 pound bone-in leg of lamb, trimmed
- Black pepper powder to taste
- 5 cups cold water
- 1 medium onion, finely chopped
- 2 large cloves garlic, minced
- ¼ cup tomato sauce
- ½ tablespoon red wine vinegar
- 2 ½ teaspoons kosher salt, divided
- 2 tablespoons extra-virgin olive oil
- 2 bay leaves
- 1 medium Cubanelle or Anaheim peppers, finely chopped
- 1 large tomato, deseeded, finely chopped
- A pinch ground cloves

Instructions:

1. Add about 1 ½ teaspoons salt and about ½ teaspoon pepper powder into a bowl and stir.
2. Rub this over the lamb.
3. Place a heavy pot over medium heat. Add ½ tablespoon oil. When the oil is heated, place the lamb in the pot.
4. Cook until brown on all the sides. Turn off the heat.

5. Transfer the lamb into the slow cooker.
6. Add bay leaves. Pour water into the slow cooker.
7. Cover the pot and cook on low for 8 to 9 hours or on high for 4 to 5 hours or until the meat is coming of the bones.
8. Switch off the cooker.
9. Remove lamb with a pair of tongs and place on your cutting board. Let it cool for a while. Shred the meat with a pair of forks until it is fine.
10. Add it back into the slow cooker.
11. Place a skillet over medium heat. Add 1-½ tablespoons of oil. When the oil is heated, add onion and Cubanelle peppers and until onions are translucent.
12. Add garlic and sauté for a few seconds until fragrant.
13. Add tomato sauce, tomatoes, cloves, remaining salt and pepper to taste.
14. Mix until well combined.
15. Cover the pot and cook on low for 1-½ hours or on high for 45 minutes.
16. Taste and adjust the seasoning if necessary.
17. Uncover and cook on high for a few minutes until the soup is reduced as per your liking.

Slow Cooker Low Carb

Hearty Chicken Stew

Makes: 8 servings

Carbs per serving: 4.9 grams

Ingredients:

- 2 pounds chicken breasts, skinless, boneless, rinsed, chopped into bite size pieces
- 2 medium carrots, sliced into rounds
- ½ red medium bell pepper, chopped into 1 inch squares
- ½ green bell pepper, chopped into 1 inch squares
- 2 stalks celery, chopped
- 12 fresh mushrooms, sliced
- 1 large ripe red tomato, chopped
- 2 cloves garlic, sliced
- ¼ cup low carb tomato sauce
- 4 tablespoons butter, unsalted
- 2 bay leaves, crumbled
- 2 sticks cinnamon
- 4 teaspoons whole peppercorns
- 2 teaspoons white pepper powder
- Salt to taste
- 6 cups water
- 2 tablespoons cooking oil

Instructions:

1. Place chicken pieces in a bowl and season with salt. Set aside for a while.
2. Place a skillet over medium heat. Add oil and butter. When butter melts, add the whole spices. Sauté for about 8-10 seconds and add garlic. Sauté until the garlic is aromatic.

3. Add onions and sauté until it is light brown. Transfer into the slow cooker.
4. Add tomatoes and stir.
5. Add tomato paste, celery, chicken, mushrooms, carrot, water and salt and mix until well combined.
6. Cover the pot. Cook on low for 4 to 5 hours or on high for 2 to 2 ½ hours.
7. Add the bell peppers during the last 15 minutes of cooking.
8. Ladle into soup bowls and serve hot.

Gruyere – Bacon Dip

Makes: 8 servings (without serving options)

Carbs per serving: 1.7 grams

Ingredients:

- ¼ cup onion, chopped
- ½ cup Gruyere cheese, shredded
- ½ teaspoon Worcestershire sauce
- Freshly ground pepper to taste
- 1 tablespoon green onion, thinly sliced
- Cooking spray
- ¼ cup canola mayonnaise
- ¼ teaspoon dry mustard
- 4 ounces fat free cream cheese, softened
- 2 center cut bacon slices

Instructions:

1. Grease the inside of the slow cooker by spraying with cooking spray.
2. Place a nonstick skillet over medium high heat. Spray with cooking spray. Add bacon and cook until crisp.
3. Remove bacon with a slotted spoon and place on a plate lined with paper towels.
4. Add onions into the skillet and sauté until translucent. Turn off heat.
5. Transfer the cooked onion into the slow cooker.
6. Add cheese, Worcestershire sauce, pepper, mayonnaise, mustard and cream cheese and mix well.
7. Cover the pot and cook on low for 50-60 minutes or on high for 25 to 30 minutes. Stir after 45 minutes of cooking on Low or 20 minutes of cooking on High.

8. Sprinkle bacon and green onions on top and serve with vegetable sticks or turkey burgers.

Hot Cheesy Roasted Brussels Sprout Dip

Makes: 8 servings

Carbs per serving: 12 grams

Ingredients:

- 2 pounds Brussels sprouts, trimmed, quartered
- Salt to taste
- Black pepper powder to taste
- 1 teaspoon fresh thyme, chopped
- ½ cup sour cream
- 1 ½ cups Mozzarella cheese, shredded
- 2 tablespoons olive oil
- 4 cloves garlic, unpeeled
- 8 ounces cream cheese, at room temperature
- ½ cup mayonnaise
- ½ cup parmesan cheese, grated

Instructions:

1. Add Brussels sprouts, salt, pepper, thyme, sour cream, mozzarella cheese, olive oil, garlic, cream cheese, mayonnaise and Parmesan cheese into the slow cooker.
2. Cover the pot and cook on low for 2 to 4 hours on high for 1 to 2 hours or until the mixture is melted.
3. Stir and serve hot.

Arianna Brooks

Grain Free Granola

Makes: 6 servings

Carbs per serving: 8.7 grams

Ingredients:

- 3 tablespoons coconut oil
- ¼ cup walnuts
- ¼ cup almonds
- ¼ cup hazelnuts
- ¼ cup pecans
- ½ cup shredded coconut, unsweetened
- ½ cup pumpkin seeds
- ½ cup sunflower seeds
- ½ teaspoon vanilla stevia
- ½ teaspoon vanilla extract
- ½ teaspoon ground cinnamon
- ¼ teaspoon swerve sweetener or any other low carb sweetener of your choice
- ½ teaspoon salt

Instructions:

1. Add coconut oil into the slow cooker.
2. Set the slow cooker on low. In a while the coconut oil will melt.
3. Add vanilla stevia and vanilla extract and stir.
4. Add walnuts, almonds, hazelnuts, pecans, coconut, sunflower seeds and pumpkin seeds. Stir until the nuts and seeds are well coated with the mixture in the pot.
5. Add swerve, salt and cinnamon into a bowl and stir. Dust all over the nut mixture.

6. Cover the pot and continue cooking on low for 2 hours or until brown and you get a whiff of the toasted mixture.
7. Stir once every half hour.
8. Transfer on to a baking sheet and spread it evenly. Cool completely. Chop or break into pieces.
9. Transfer into an airtight container.

Arianna Brooks

Cranberry-Citrus Meatballs

Makes: 16 servings (2 meatballs per serving)

Carbs per serving: 8 grams

Ingredients:

- 1 pound ground pork
- ¼ cup dried cranberries, finely chopped
- 1/8 teaspoon black pepper powder
- ½ can (from a 14.5 ounce can) whole berry cranberry sauce
- 2 tablespoons orange juice
- 1 egg, lightly beaten
- ½ cup cooked long grain brown rice
- ½ teaspoon salt or to taste
- 1 to 2 teaspoons olive oil
- 3 tablespoons low carb ketchup
- 1 tablespoon lime juice

Instructions:

1. Add pork, cranberries, pepper, salt, egg and rice into a bowl and mix until well combined.
2. Divide the mixture into 32 equal portions. Form balls of each portion.
3. Place a large skillet over medium heat. Add oil and swirl the pan. When the oil is heated, add meatballs and cook until brown on all the sides. Do not cook the meatballs thoroughly. Just enough for them not to disintegrate.
4. Remove the meatballs and place in the slow cooker.
5. Add ketchup, cranberry sauce, lime juice and orange juice into a bowl and stir. Transfer into the slow cooker. Stir until the mixture coats the meatballs well.

6. Cover the pot and cook on low for 3-4 hours or on high for 1 ½ -2 hours.
7. When done, stir once again. Transfer onto a serving platter. Insert toothpicks in each meatball and serve.

Arianna Brooks

Italian Cocktail Meatballs

Makes: 12 servings (2 meatballs per serving)

Carbs per serving: 6 grams

Ingredients:

- 2 packages (12 ounces each with 12 meatballs in each package) frozen cooked turkey meatballs, thawed
- ¼ teaspoon crushed red pepper
- A handful fresh snipped basil (optional)
- 1 cup bottled roasted red and / or yellow sweet peppers, drained, cut into 1 inch piece
- 2 cups bottled low sodium pasta sauce

Instructions:

1. Place meatballs in the slow cooker. Scatter roasted peppers over the meatballs.
2. Spoon pasta sauce over the meatballs. Dust with crushed red pepper.
3. Cover the pot and cook on low for 4-5 hours or on high for 2 – 2 ½ hours.
4. Carefully remove the fat floating on top and discard it. Stir and transfer onto a serving platter.
5. Sprinkle basil. Insert toothpicks in each meatball and serve.

Slow Cooker Low Carb

Apricot-Honey Mustard Sausage Bites

Makes: 16 servings (2 sausage slices and 1 piece apricot)

Carbs per serving: 7 grams

Ingredients:

- 1/3 cup apricot preserve or sugar-free apricot preserves
- ½ small onion, chopped
- ½ tablespoon water
- 1 package (12 ounces with 8 links) apple flavored, cooked chicken sausage links
- 4 dried apricots, quartered
- 1 ½ tablespoons honey mustard
- ¼ teaspoon snipped fresh thyme

Instructions:

1. Place sausage link on your cutting board. Cut on the bias into 8 slices.
2. Repeat the previous step with the remaining sausage links. You should have 32 sausage slices in all.
3. Add dried apricots, apricot preserves, honey mustard, onion and water into the slow cooker and stir.
4. Add sausages and stir until the mixture is well coated on the sausages.
5. Cover the pot and cook on low for 3-4 hours or on high for 1 ½ - 2 hours.
6. Add thyme and stir.
7. Serve.

Arianna Brooks

Slow-Cooker Buffalo Chicken Dip

Makes: 16 servings

Carbs per serving: 2 grams

Ingredients:

- 1 chopped large onion
- 1 pound trimmed chicken breasts (boneless and skinless)
- 1 cup low-sodium chicken broth
- 8 ounces reduced-fat cream cheese
- 3 tablespoons hot sauce
- 1 finely chopped large jalapeño pepper,
- Sliced scallions, to garnish
- 1/4 cup blue cheese (crumbled) + more for garnishing

Instructions:

1. Pour the chicken broth into the slow cooker. Add the onion and jalapeno pepper to the broth.
2. Place the chicken on the top and mix well.
3. Cover the cooker and cook on high for 2.5 hours.
4. Once the cooking cycle is over, transfer the cooked chicken to a plate and shred it using 2 forks.
5. Place an aluminum foil over the shredded chicken and set aside.
6. Slowly drain the liquid from the slow cooker, add the cream cheese and 1/4 cup blue cheese into the slow cooker.
7. Mix well and add the hot sauce to it. Whisk the mixture using an immersion blender until smooth.

8. Cover the cooker and cook for 20 minutes until the contents are heated through.
9. After 20 minutes, add the shredded chicken to the slow cooker and mix well gently.
10. Top it with blue cheese and scallions.
11. Transfer to a plate and serve warm!

Arianna Brooks

Cheese Fondue with Fennel & Tomatoes

Makes: 12 servings

Carbs per serving: 6 grams

Ingredients:

- 3½ cups shredded Swiss or Emmentaler cheese (around 10 ounces)
- 1 teaspoon gently crushed fennel seeds
- 2 cups shredded Gruyère or Comté cheese (around 6 ounces)
- 14 ounces unsalted diced tomatoes, drained well (1 can)
- 1 cup onion (diced)
- 1 1/2 tablespoons extra-virgin olive oil
- 2 cups fennel (diced)
- 1 1/4 cups white wine (light, fruity), you can use dry Riesling
- 1/4 teaspoon salt
- 2 tablespoons all-purpose flour
- Freshly ground pepper, to taste
- 1/4 teaspoon cayenne pepper

Instructions:

1. Pour hot boiling water into a slow cooker and set aside to let it warm
2. Heat oil over medium heat in a large skillet and add the diced fennel to it.
3. Stir the fennel in the oil and add the chopped onion.
4. Sauté for 10 minutes as you stir often until the contents turn translucent

5. Add the tomatoes, pepper and salt to the contents in the skillet.
6. Continue to cook for 4 minutes as you stir once in a while. Wait until all the liquid evaporates and turn off the heat. Set it aside.
7. Take a medium-sized bowl and combine the crushed fennel seeds, Swiss cheese, Gruyere cheese, all-purpose flour and cayenne pepper. Mix them well until the contents blend. Set it aside.
8. Heat a heavy-bottomed medium-sized saucepan over medium heat and add wine when hot. Let it cook until it gets heated through.
9. Add the cheese-flour mixture to the pan one handful at a time. Keep stirring until it melts before you add the next handful.
10. Remove from heat and set aside.
11. Drain the slow cooker and pat dry. Pour the cheese mixture into the slow cooker and add the cooked vegetable mixture into it.
12. Stir well until combined. Cover the cooker and cook on high for 10 minutes.
13. Set it on warm before you serve.
14. Transfer to a bowl and serve with your favorite bread.
15. Add one or two teaspoons of flour to the slow cooker if the fondue begins to separate. Keep the cooker set to warm always.

Arianna Brooks

Bourbon-Glazed Cocktail Sausages

Makes: 12 servings

Carbs per serving: 7 grams

Ingredients:

- 16 ounces smoked turkey sausage or smoked Polish sausage (lightly cooked), cut into 1-inch slices
- 1 tablespoon bourbon
- 1 teaspoon crushed quick-cooking tapioca
- 3 tablespoons pure maple syrup
- 1/3 cup apricot preserves (low-sugar)

Instructions:

1. Place the smoked sausage slices in the slow cooker (preferably 1 1/2 quart cooker).
2. Add bourbon, crushed tapioca, maple syrup and apricot preserves to the cooker.
3. Cover and cook on low for 4 hours (in case you don't find any heat setting available, just cook for 4 hours)
4. Transfer the cooked sausages to a plate.
5. You can insert wooden toothpicks into the sausages and serve!

Slow Cooker Low Carb

Slow-Cooker Chicken Enchilada Dip

Makes: 12 servings

Carbs per serving: 11 grams

Ingredients:

- 1 pound chicken breast (boneless and skinless)
- 5 ounces rinsed black beans (1 can)
- 2 cups chopped fresh tomatoes (2 medium ones should do)
- 1 cup fresh or frozen corn (thawed if you are using frozen corn)
- 1 cup onion (chopped)
- 1 stemmed fresh jalapeño pepper
- 2 garlic cloves
- 8 ounces reduced-fat cream cheese
- 2 tablespoons fresh cilantro (chopped)
- 1 cup sharp cheddar cheese (shredded)
- 1 tablespoon chili powder
- 2 tablespoons scallions (sliced)
- 1 teaspoon ground cumin
- 3/4 teaspoon salt

Instructions:

1. Combine the tomatoes, onion, jalapeno pepper, garlic, cumin, chili powder and salt in a high-speed blender. Blend on high for 60 seconds until it gets a smooth puree consistency.
2. Pour this tomato-onion-pepper sauce into the slow cooker and place the chicken into it.
3. Coat the meat with the sauce by stirring using a spatula.

4. Cover the cooker and cook on high for 3 hours or on low heat for 6 hours.
5. After the cooking cycle, remove the cooked chicken and transfer to a big plate. Shred the meat using two forks and put them back into the sauce in the slow cooker.
6. Add the cheddar cheese, cream cheese, corn and beans to the mixture in the cooker.
7. Stir well until combined. Cover the cooker and cook on high for 15 minutes until the cheese melts and the sauce gets heated through.
8. Transfer to a bowl and top the dip with cilantro and scallions.
9. Serve warm and enjoy!

Middle Eastern Lamb Stew

Makes: 8 servings

Carbs per serving: 12 grams

Ingredients:

- 2 1/2 pounds deboned & trimmed lamb shoulder chops (cut into 1-inch chunks)
- 6 ounces baby spinach
- 3/4 cup reduced-sodium chicken broth
- 1 large onion (chopped)
- 4 minced garlic cloves
- 15 ounces rinsed chickpeas (1 can)
- 28 ounces diced tomatoes (1 can)
- 1 tablespoon ground coriander
- 1/4 teaspoon cayenne pepper
- 4 teaspoons cumin (ground)
- Freshly ground pepper, to taste
- 1 tablespoon olive oil
- 1/4 teaspoon salt
- Nonstick cooking spray

Instructions:

1. Grease the insides of the slow cooker with a nonstick cooking spray and place the lamb chunks in it
2. Take a small bowl and mix the oil, cumin, cayenne, coriander, pepper and salt together.
3. Add this oil-spice paste to the cooker and toss to coat the meat well with it.
4. Add the onions over the coated meat and set the cooker aside.

5. Heat a medium-sized saucepan over medium-high heat and add the tomatoes to the hot pan.
6. Pour the broth and add the garlic to the pan. Let it simmer until the tomatoes become mushy and break. Stir well until the liquid gets a thick or sauce-like consistency
7. Pour this sauce mixture over the onions in the cooker and cover it.
8. Cook on high for 3.5 hours or on low heat for 6 hours until the meat becomes soft and tender.
9. Once the cooking cycle is over, skim the visible fat from the surface of the stew.
10. Take a small bowl and place 1/2-cup chickpeas in it. Using a fork, mash the chickpeas thoroughly.
11. Add the mashed chickpeas the stew and mix well. Now, add the remaining whole chickpeas and mix well until combined
12. Add the spinach, cover the cooker and cook on high for 5 minutes until the spinach wilts.
13. Transfer to a serving bowl and enjoy!

Low Carb Chipotle Cauliflower Cheese

Makes: 4 servings

Carbs per serving: 11 grams

Ingredients:

- 1 medium cauliflower (cut into florets)
- 2 cups cheddar cheese (shredded)
- 1/2 cup mayonnaise
- 4 ounces softened cream cheese
- 1/2 cup almond milk (unsweetened)
- 2 teaspoons onion powder
- Black pepper, to taste
- 1 teaspoon chipotle powder
- Chipotle flakes, to garnish
- Nonstick cooking spray

Instructions:

1. Take a large bowl and combine the cheddar cheese, mayonnaise, cream cheese, onion powder, black pepper and chipotle powder. Mix well until blended.
2. Grease the insides of a slow cooker with the nonstick cooking spray.
3. Place the cauliflower florets in the cooker and add the cheese cream mixture to it.
4. Pour the almond milk and stir the contents until the ingredients are well combined.
5. Cover the cooker and cook on low heat for 3 hours until the florets become soft and tender. If you like the cauliflower to be a bit crunchy, you can cook for 2.5 hours.

6. Transfer to a bowl and garnish with chipotle flakes. Serve and enjoy!

Slow Cooker Lamb with Thyme

Makes: 2 servings

Carbs per serving: 3 grams

Ingredients:

- 2 bone-in lamb shoulder chops
- 1/4 cup fresh thyme sprigs + extra thyme leaves
- 1 cup chicken broth
- 1 teaspoon garlic paste
- 1/2 cup red wine
- Salt and pepper, to taste

Instructions:

1. Trim the meat if necessary and wash.
2. Place the trimmed lamb shoulder chops in a slow cooker.
3. Pour the chicken broth and add the thyme sprigs, garlic paste and red wine into the cooker.
4. Stir until combined thoroughly. Cover and cook on high for 3 hours or on low heat for 6 hours.
5. Once the cooking cycle is over, remove the meat and chop them into smaller chunks if needed.
6. Transfer to a serving plate and pour a large spoonful of the liquid from the cooker over the chopped meat.
7. Season with pepper and salt if required. Serve hot and enjoy!

Arianna Brooks

Mustard Cocktail Sausages

Makes: 6 servings

Carbs per serving: 2 grams (excluding sugar alcohols)

Ingredients:

- 14 ounces cocktail sausages
- 3 tablespoon wholegrain mustard
- 1 tablespoon low carb sweetener Swerve
- Nonstick cooking spray

Instructions:

1. Grease the inside of the slow cooker with a nonstick cooking spray.
2. Place the cocktail sausages in the cooker and add in the mustard and sweetener.
3. Toss to coat the sausages and cover the cooker.
4. Cook on low heat for 5 hours or on high for 3 hours
5. Stir once halfway through the cooking time.
6. Once the cooking cycle is complete, transfer the sausages to a plate.
7. Serve hot and enjoy!

Low Carb Buffalo Almonds

Makes: 8 servings

Carbs per serving: 7 grams

Ingredients:

- 10 ounces whole almonds (raw)
- 2 tablespoons hot sauce
- 4 tablespoons melted butter (unsalted)
- Salt, to taste
- Nonstick cooking spray

Instructions:

1. Grease the inside of the slow cooker with a nonstick cooking spray
2. Add the almonds, hot sauce and melted butter into the cooker.
3. Stir until the almonds are coated with the sauce and butter
4. Cover and cook on low heat for 2 hours.
5. Line a baking sheet with parchment paper and spread the cooked nuts over it
6. Sprinkle with salt and let it sit for some time allowing it to cook
7. Transfer to a bowl and serve!

Arianna Brooks

Low Carb BBQ Party Sausages

Makes: 8 servings

Carbs per serving: 4 grams

Ingredients:

- 28 ounces mini sausages (2 packages)
- 8 ounces canned tomato sauce (please don't use ketchup)
- 1 teaspoon dry mustard powder
- 2 tablespoons white wine vinegar
- 1 teaspoon paprika
- 1/2 teaspoon garlic paste
- 2 tablespoons sugar-free sweetening syrup (Da Vinci or similar)
- Salt and pepper, to taste
- Nonstick cooking spray

Instructions:

1. Grease the insides of the slow cooker with a nonstick cooking spray
2. Add the tomato sauce, mustard powder, white wine vinegar, paprika, garlic paste, syrup, salt and pepper into the slow cooker.
3. Mix them well until the flavors blend. Add the mini sausages and stir to coat with the sauce.
4. Cover and cook on high for 3 hours and on low heat for 5 hours. Stir once halfway through the cooking time.
5. Transfer to a plate and serve the sausages hot!

Chapter Nine - Desserts

Pumpkin Pie Pudding

Makes: 12 servings

Carbs per serving: 8 grams

Ingredients:

For pumpkin pudding

- 2 cans (15 ounces each) pureed pumpkin
- 4 eggs
- 2 teaspoons pumpkin pie spice
- 1 cup heavy whipping cream
- 2 teaspoons vanilla extract
- 1 ½ cups erythritol or swerve or truvia or splenda

For topping

- 1 cup heavy whipping cream

Instructions:

1. Grease the inside of the slow cooker with a little oil or butter.
2. Add eggs into a large bowl and whisk well.
3. Add swerve and whisk until it dissolves.
4. Add pumpkin puree, pumpkin pie spice, vanilla extract and cream and whisk until well combined. Pour into the slow cooker.
5. Cover the pot and cook on low for 6 to 7 hours or until set. Switch off the cooker and let it cool.
6. Serve warm or cold topped with heavy cream.

Arianna Brooks

Chocolate Truffle Crème Brulee

Makes: 2 servings

Carbs per serving: 10 grams

Ingredients:

- 1 cup heavy cream
- 3 tablespoons sukrin or monk fruit sweetener or swerve, divided
- ¼ teaspoon stevia
- 3 egg yolks
- 1.75 oz. 80 to 90% dark chocolate
- 1 tablespoon good brandy
- Whipped cream to top (optional)
- Extra sweetener to sprinkle

Instructions:

1. Add yolks and ½ tablespoon granulated sweetener into a bowl and whisk until the sweetener is dissolved completely.
2. Add cream, stevia and remaining sweetener into a saucepan. Place the saucepan over medium heat until bubbles are slightly visible along the edges of the saucepan. Remove from heat.
3. Whisking simultaneously, pour egg yolk mixture in a very thin stream. Whisk constantly until all of it is added.
4. Add chocolate chips and whisk until chocolate melts.
5. Add brandy and whisk until well combined. Pour the mixture equally into 2 ramekins.

6. Pour about 2 to 3 cups water in the slow cooker. Place the ramekins in it. The sides of the ramekins should be covered with water up to half its length.
7. Cover the pot and cook on low for 1 ½ -2 hours or until the custard sets and jiggles very slightly in the center.
8. When done, cool completely and place in the refrigerator for a few hours to chill.
9. Sprinkle granulated sweetener on top. Caramelize the sprinkled sweetener with a culinary torch.
10. If you do not want to caramelize, then serve topped with whipped cream.

Arianna Brooks

Mocha Pudding Cake

Makes: 12 servings

Carbs per serving: 7.36 grams

Ingredients:

- 1 ½ cups butter, chopped into chunks
- 1 cup heavy cream
- 2 teaspoons vanilla extract
- 2/3 cup almond flour
- 10 large eggs
- 4 oz. chocolate, unsweetened, finely chopped
- 4 tablespoons instant coffee crystals
- 8 tablespoons cocoa powder, unsweetened
- ¼ teaspoon salt
- 1 1/3 cups granulated erythritol or stevia
- Cooking spray or butter to grease

To serve (optional)

- Low carb ice cream
- Whipped cream

Instructions:

1. Grease the inside of the slow cooker by with cooking spray or softened butter.
2. Add butter and chocolate into a saucepan. Place the saucepan over low heat. Stir occasionally. Heat until the mixture is melted and well combined. Alternately, add butter and chocolate into a heatproof bowl. Place the bowl in a double boiler and melt the chocolate.
3. Turn off the heat and cool.

4. Add cream, vanilla and coffee into the melted chocolate bowl. Whisk well.
5. Add almond flour, cocoa, and salt into another bowl and stir.
6. Add eggs into a bowl and beat until slightly they become thick.
7. Add erythritol and beat until the mixture turns light yellow in color. (Best to use an electric mixer)
8. Set the speed of the mixer to the lowest speed and add the chocolate mixture.
9. Add the almond flour mixture and beat until well combined.
10. Set the speed of the mixer to medium speed and add the cream mixture. Beat until well combined.
11. Pour the batter into the slow cooker.
12. Cover the top of the slow cooker pot with paper towels.
13. Cover the pot and cook on low for 2-3 hours.
14. When the cake pudding is ready, the center should be soft and moist and yet firm to touch.
15. Garnish with whipped cream or ice cream if desired.

Arianna Brooks

Slow Cooker Baby Bok Choy Brownies

Makes: 16 servings

Carbs per serving: 10.33 grams

Ingredients:

- 2 packages (5 count each) Jade Asian Greens Baby Shanghai Bok Choy, trimmed
- 1 teaspoon salt
- 1 cup cocoa powder
- 2 teaspoons baking powder
- 4 large eggs
- 2 teaspoons vanilla extract
- 4 tablespoons water
- 2 cups almond flour
- 1 cup granulated swerve or erythritol
- 1 teaspoon espresso powder (optional)
- 2/3 cup coconut oil, melted
- 2/3 cup dark chocolate chips (optional)
- Cooking spray

Instructions:

1. Grease the inside of the slow cooker with cooking spray. Preferably use a large cooker.
2. Separate the leaves of the Bok Choy from the stems. Use the leaves for some other recipe. Chop the stems into small pieces.
3. Place saucepan with water over medium heat. Add Bok Choy stems and salt into the saucepan.
4. When it begins to boil, lower the heat and simmer for 5 minutes.
5. Turn off the heat. Cool slightly and add into a blender.

6. Blend for 40-50 seconds until smooth.
7. Add cocoa powder, baking powder almond flour, swerve and espresso powder into a bowl and stir.
8. Add pureed Bok Choy, eggs, vanilla extract, water and coconut oil into another bowl and mix well.
9. Pour Bok Choy mixture into the bowl of almond flour mixture. Mix until well combined.
10. Add chocolate chips and fold.
11. Spoon the batter into the slow cooker.
12. Cover the pot and cook on low for 4 hours or a toothpick when inserted in the center comes out clean.
13. Cool for a while. Slice and serve.

Arianna Brooks

Blueberry Lemon Custard Cake

Makes: 6 servings

Carbs per serving: 4 grams

Ingredients:

- ¼ cup coconut flour
- ¼ cup swerve sweetener
- 3 eggs, separated
- 3 tablespoons lemon juice
- 1 teaspoon lemon zest
- ½ teaspoon lemon liquid stevia
- ¼ teaspoon salt
- ¼ cup fresh blueberries
- 1 cup heavy cream
- Cooking spray

To serve (optional)

- Whipped cream, sugar-free

Instructions:

1. Add whites into a mixing bowl. Beat with an electric mixer until stiff peaks are formed. Set aside.
2. Add yolks into another bowl and whisk well.
3. Add coconut flour, swerve, lemon juice, lemon zest, lemon stevia, salt, blueberries and heavy cream and beat until well combined.
4. Add whites, a tablespoon at a time and fold gently each time until all of it is added.
5. Grease the inside of the slow cooker by spraying with cooking spray.

6. Spoon the batter into the slow cooker.
7. Scatter blueberries on top. Press lightly so that the blueberries are slightly embedded in the batter.
8. Cover the pot and cook on low for 3 hours a knitting needle or a knife when inserted in the center comes out clean.
9. Uncover and cool for an hour. Chill for 2-8 hours.
10. Chop into 6 equal portions and serve with whipped cream if using.

Arianna Brooks

Healthy Chocolate Muffins

Makes: 5 servings

Carbs per serving: 5 grams

Ingredients:

Dry ingredients

- 6 tablespoons coconut flour
- 2 tablespoons cocoa powder
- ¼ teaspoon instant coffee granules
- 1/8 teaspoon salt
- ¼ cup Sukrin 1 or swerve, granulated
- ½ tablespoon baking powder
- 1/8 teaspoon xanthan gum
- 2.5 ounces zucchini, grated

Wet ingredients

- 3 large eggs
- ¼ teaspoon stevia drops
- ¼ teaspoon vanilla extract
- 2 tablespoons sugar free chocolate chips

Melting ingredients

- 0.5 ounce baking chocolate, unsweetened, slivered
- 2 ounces butter or ghee

Instructions:

1. Grease 5 muffin cups with cooking spray and set aside.
2. Sprinkle a little salt over the zucchini and place in a colander. Set aside for a while.

Slow Cooker Low Carb

3. Add rest of the dry ingredients into a bowl and stir.
4. Add melting ingredients (butter and baking chocolate) into a microwave safe bowl. Microwave for a few seconds until it melts. Give increments of 30 seconds and whisk before each increment. Alternately, add chocolate and butter into a heatproof bowl and melt in a double boiler.
5. Add wet ingredients into another bowl and whisk well. Pour into the bowl of dry ingredients. Mix with an electric hand mixer until well combined and free from lumps.
6. Add melted chocolate and butter mixture and mix until well combined.
7. Squeeze the zucchini of excess moisture and add into the batter. Beat until well combined
8. Mix well and spoon into the prepared greased muffin cups. Fill up to ¾ the mold. Sprinkle chocolate chips on top.
9. Place a layer of crumpled aluminum foil at the bottom of the cooker (this step can be avoided if your cooking pot is ceramic). Place the muffin cups inside the slow cooker, over the aluminum foil.
10. Cover the pot and cook on high for 2 to 3 hours or until a toothpick or knitting needle when inserted in the center of the muffins comes out clean.
11. Let it cool in the cooker for a while.
12. Cool slightly. Run a knife around the edges. Invert onto a plate and serve.

Arianna Brooks

Slow-Cooker Chai Apple Butter

Makes: 28 servings

Carbs per serving: 14 grams

Ingredients:

- 16 cups McIntosh or Ananas Reinette apples (peeled and sliced into ½ inch thick pieces); around 5 pounds (*Note: if you don't get these apples, you can use any other juicy-type apple*)
- 2 teaspoons ground cinnamon
- 2/3 cup dark brown sugar (tightly packed)
- 2 teaspoons ground cardamom
- 1 tablespoon vanilla extract
- 2 teaspoons ground turmeric
- 2 teaspoons coriander (ground)
- 1/2 teaspoon salt

Instructions:

1. Combine the apples, cinnamon, brown sugar, cardamom, vanilla extract, turmeric, coriander and salt in a slow cooker.
2. Mix well until combined.
3. Cover the cooker and cook on high for 5 hours. Stir occasionally once or twice in between the cooking cycle.
4. After 5 hours, open the cooker and stir the contents open. Partially close the cooker and continue to cook for 2 more hours until the apples are completely mashed or broken
5. Transfer the contents of the slow cooker to a food processor after 2 hours.

6. Pulse it once until you get a smooth and creamy mixture.
7. Transfer to a bowl and get ready to serve.

Arianna Brooks

Slow Cooker Low Carb Maple Custard

Makes: 6 servings

Carbs per serving: 2 grams

Ingredients:

- 1 teaspoon maple extract
- 1/2 cup whole milk
- 2 egg yolks (lightly beaten)
- 1 cup heavy cream
- 2 eggs (beaten)
- 1/2 teaspoon cinnamon
- 1/4 cup sugar-free brown sugar substitute like Sukrin Gold
- 1/4 teaspoon salt
- Sugar-free whipped cream, as desired

Instructions:

1. Combine the maple extract, beaten yolk, heavy cream, beaten eggs, whole milk, cinnamon, sukrin gold and salt in a high-speed blender.
2. Blend on medium-high for 45 seconds until completely smooth and creamy
3. Grease 6 ramekins (4-ounce capacity) and pour the blended mixture evenly into each of them. Ensure you fill only 3/4th of the ramekin.
4. Place 4 ramekins to the bottom of the slow cooker and the remaining two against one side of the cooker.
5. Cover and cook on high for 2 hours until the center is set but a bit jiggly.

6. Remove from the cooker and let it cool for an hour at room temperature.
7. After the 1-hour cooling process, refrigerate it for 2 hours and let it chill.
8. Serve the custards with sugar-free whipped cream and enjoy!

Arianna Brooks

Slow Cooker Low Carb Mint Chocolate Cake

Makes: 8 servings

Carbs per serving: 8 grams

Ingredients:

- 1/3 cup mini chocolate chips (low carb)
- 1/3 cup cocoa powder (unsweetened)
- 2/3 cup almond milk (unsweetened)
- 3 beaten eggs
- 6 tablespoons + extra melted and cooled butter (unsalted)
- 1 cup almond flour
- 1/2 teaspoon peppermint extract
- 1 1/2 teaspoons baking powder
- 1/2 cup sweetener (like xylitol)
- 1/4 teaspoon salt

Instructions:

1. Take a large bowl and combine the cocoa powder, almond flour, baking powder, sweetener and salt in it. Mix well.
2. Add the almond milk, beaten eggs, melted butter, peppermint extract and chocolate chips into the bowl.
3. Mix well until the contents are well incorporated.
4. Grease the inside of a slow cooker with the melted butter and pour the batter in it.
5. Cover the cooker and let it cook over low heat for 3 hours.
6. Turn off the heat and leave the cake in the cooker to cool for 30 minutes.

7. Transfer to a plate and serve warm.

Arianna Brooks

Low Carb Chocolate Fondue

Makes: 8 servings

Carbs per serving: 12 grams

Ingredients:

- 1 cup heavy cream
- 2 30 ounces low carb Dark Chocolate bars
- Nonstick cooking spray

Instructions:

1. Grease the insides of the slow cooker with a nonstick cooking spray
2. Place the dark chocolate bars in the cooker and add the heavy cream over it.
3. Cover and cook on low heat for 1.5 hours.
4. Transfer to a plate and serve warm.

Slow Cooker Dark Chocolate Cake

Makes: 10 servings

Carbs per serving: 8.42 grams

Ingredients:

- 1 cup + 2 tablespoons almond flour
- 3 tablespoons whey protein powder (unflavored)
- 3 large eggs (beaten)
- 1/2 cup cocoa powder
- 2/3 cup almond milk (unsweetened)
- 6 tablespoons melted butter
- 1 1/2 teaspoon baking powder
- 3/4 teaspoon vanilla extract
- 1/2 cup Swerve Granular
- 1/3 cup chocolate chips (sugar-free)
- 1/4 teaspoon salt
- Nonstick cooking spray

Instructions:

1. Grease the inside of the slow cooker with a nonstick cooking spray
2. Take a medium bowl and whisk together cocoa powder, almond flour, baking powder, whey protein powder and sweetener in it.
3. Add the beaten eggs, melted butter, vanilla extract and unsweetened almond milk into the dry mixture of the bowl
4. Mix thoroughly until the ingredients are well blended.
5. Add the chocolate chips into the mixture.

6. Pour this mixture into the greased inside of the cooker and cover.
7. Cook on low heat for 2.5 hours until the cake is completely set
8. Turn off the cooker and let it cool for 30 minutes.
9. Cut the cake into small pieces and transfer to a plate.
10. Serve warm and enjoy.

Slow Cooker Low Carb

Slow Cooker Raspberry Cream Cheese Cake

Makes: 12 servings

Carbs per serving: 6.95 grams

Ingredients:

For the cake batter

- 1 1/4 almond flour
- 3 large eggs (beaten)
- 1/4 cup protein powder
- 6 tablespoons melted butter
- 1/4 cup coconut flour
- 1/2 teaspoon vanilla extract
- 1 1/2 teaspoon baking powder
- 2/3 cup water
- 1/2 cup swerve sweetener
- 1/4 tsp salt
- Nonstick cooking spray

For the filling

- 2 tablespoons whipping cream
- 8 ounces cream cheese
- 1 1/2 cup fresh raspberries
- 1/3 cup Swerve Sweetener (powdered)
- 1 large egg (beaten)

Instructions:

1. Grease the ceramic insert of the slow cooker with a nonstick cooking spray.

407

2. To prepare the cake batter, take a large bowl. Combine the coconut flour, almond flour, salt, and sweetener, baking powder and protein powder in the bowl. Mix thoroughly.
3. Now, add the beaten eggs, water and melted water into the bowl. Stir thoroughly until completely incorporated. Set this aside and start making the filling.
4. Take another bowl and beat together the sweetener and cream cheese until smooth. Add in the eggs and whipping cream to the mixture and stir until combined thoroughly.
5. Spread two-thirds of the cake batter to the bottom of the cooker and smoothen it in the top using a spatula.
6. Now pour the cheese cream mixture and spread evenly. Sprinkle the raspberries over this layer.
7. Dot the remaining cake batter over the cheese mixture (fillings) in small spoonfuls such that they peek through
8. Cover the cooker and let it cook on low for 4 hours until the edges turn golden brown.
9. The filling will barely set in the middle and might jiggle slightly when you shake.
10. Turn off the cooker and remove the insert. Let it cool at room temperature for an hour.
11. Refrigerate it for 3 hours before you serve. Enjoy!

Flan

Makes: 10 servings

Carbs per serving: 2.1 grams

Ingredients:

- 10 eggs
- 2 cups heavy cream
- 2 cups water
- 10 packets sugar substitute or to taste
- 2 teaspoons almond extract
- ¼ teaspoon cinnamon powder
- Cooking spray

Instructions:

1. Whisk together all the ingredients except the cinnamon powder.
2. Grease a baking dish, which fits well into the slow cooker. Place it on the metal rack of the cooker.
3. Pour the whisked mixture into the baking dish. Sprinkle cinnamon powder. Cover the dish with aluminum foil.
4. Cover and cook on low for 6-7 hours or high for 2 hours or until set.
5. Can be served warm or chilled.

Arianna Brooks

Pumpkin Pie Custard

Makes: 12 servings

Carbs per serving: 7 grams

Ingredients:

- 2 cans (15 ounce each) pumpkin puree
- 1 cup 1% milk
- 8 eggs, beaten
- ½ teaspoon salt
- 1 ½ tablespoon vanilla extract
- 1 ½ tablespoon pumpkin spice
- 2 teaspoons liquid stevia or to taste
- A large pinch nutmeg powder
- Dairy free whipped cream to serve

Instructions:

1. Whisk together all the ingredients except the nutmeg powder and whipped cream.
2. Grease a baking dish that fits well into the slow cooker. Place it on the metal rack of the cooker.
3. Pour the whisked mixture into the baking dish. Sprinkle nutmeg powder. Cover the dish with aluminum foil.
4. Cover and cook on low for 6-7 hours or high for 2 hours or until set.
5. Can be served warm or chilled with dairy free whipped cream.

Carrot Pudding

Makes: 6 servings

Carbs per serving: 15 grams

Ingredients:

- 3 cups carrots, peeled, grated
- 3 cups low fat milk (1%)
- ¼ teaspoon cardamom powder
- 1 tablespoon raisins
- 2 tablespoons almond, slivered
- Stevia drops to taste

Instructions:

1. Place the carrots and milk in the slow cooker.
2. Cover and cook on low for 4-5 hours.
3. Add raisins and stir. Cook for 30 minutes more.
4. If you like it thicker, then cook for some more time.
5. Add 1-½ tablespoons almonds, stevia drops, and cardamom. Mix well.
6. Serve warm sprinkled with the remaining almonds.

Arianna Brooks

Dark Chocolate Cake

Makes: 10 servings

Carbs per serving: 11.65 grams

Ingredients:
- 1 ½ cups of almond flour
- 2/3 cup of cocoa powder
- ¾ cup of natural sweetener
- ¼ cup of whey protein powder (unflavored)
- ¼ tsp of salt
- 2 tsp of baking powder
- ½ cup of butter, melted
- ¾ cup of almond milk (unsweetened)
- 4 large eggs
- 1 tsp of vanilla extract

Instructions:
1. Grease the sides of the slow cooker.
2. In a mixing bowl, whisk the natural sweetener, almond flour, whey protein powder, cocoa powder, salt and baking powder together.
3. Add in the eggs, melted butter, vanilla extract, almond milk and stir until the ingredients are properly incorporated.
4. Pour the mixture into the slow cooker and cook for 3 hours on low settings.
5. Once done, let it cool for at least 20 minutes before cutting into pieces and serving.

Pumpkin Spice Cake

Makes: 10 servings

Carbs per serving: 10.03 grams

Ingredients:

- 1 ½ cups of raw pecans
- 1/3 cup of coconut flour
- ¾ cup of natural sweetener
- ¼ cup of whey protein powder (unflavored)
- 1 ½ tsp of ground cinnamon
- 2 tsp of baking powder
- 1 tsp of ground ginger
- ¼ tsp of salt
- ¼ tsp of ground cloves
- 1 cup of pumpkin puree
- ¼ cup of butter, melted
- 4 large eggs
- 1 tsp of vanilla extract

Instructions:

1. Line the slow cooker with parchment paper.
2. Using a food processor, grind the pecans until it becomes a coarse meal then transfer it into a mixing bowl and whisk in the natural sweetener, whey protein powder, coconut flour, baking powder, ginger, cinnamon, salt and cloves.
3. Add in the pumpkin puree, butter, eggs and vanilla extract into the mixture and stir until well combined.
4. Pour the batter into the slow cooker and cover. Cook for 3 hours on low setting.

Arianna Brooks

Carrot Cake with Cream Cheese

Makes: 12 servings

Carbs per serving: 9.5 grams

Ingredients:

- 1 ½ cups of almond flour
- ½ cup of shredded coconut
- ¾ cup of natural sweetener
- ½ cup of chopped walnuts
- 2 tsp of baking powder
- ¼ cup of whey protein powder (unflavored)
- 1 tsp of ground cinnamon
- ¼ tsp of salt
- ¼ tsp of ground cloves
- 2 cups of grated carrots
- ¼ cup of coconut oil, melted
- 4 large eggs
- 3 tbsp. of almond milk
- ½ tsp of vanilla extract
- 6 oz. of cream cheese, softened
- ¾ tsp of vanilla extract
- ½ cup of powdered natural sweetener
- ½ cup of heavy cream

Instructions:

1. Grease the sides of the slow cooker then line it with parchment paper.

2. In a mixing bowl, whisk the natural sweetener, almond flour, chopped walnuts, shredded coconut, baking powder, whey protein powder, cloves, cinnamon and salt together until properly combined.
3. Add in the eggs, carrots, almond milk, coconut oil and vanilla extract then stir until well incorporated.
4. Pour the batter into the Crockpot and cook for 3 ½ hours on low settings. Once done, let it cool completely before transferring on a serving platter.
5. To make the cream cheese frosting, beat the cream cheese together with the powdered natural sweetener until it forms a smooth mixture. Add in the vanilla extract and heavy cream and beat until properly combined. Spread the mixture over the cooled cake.

Arianna Brooks

Gingerbread

Makes: 10 servings

Carbs per serving: 8.58 grams

Ingredients:

- 2 ¼ cups of almond flour
- 2 tbsp. of coconut flour
- ¾ cup of natural sweetener
- 1 tbsp. of dark cocoa powder
- ½ tbsp. of ground cinnamon
- 1 ½ tbsp. of ground ginger
- 2 tsp of baking powder
- ¼ tsp of salt
- ½ tsp of ground cloves
- ½ cup of butter, melted
- 2/3 cup of almond milk
- 4 large eggs
- 1 tbsp. of squeezed lemon juice
- 1 tsp of vanilla extract

Instructions:

1. Grease the insides of the slow cooker.
2. In a mixing bowl, whisk the almond flour, natural sweetener, cocoa powder, coconut flour, cinnamon, ginger, baking powder, salt and cloves together. Add in the melted butter, almond milk, eggs, lemon juice and vanilla extract. Stir until all the ingredients are properly incorporated.

3. Pour the batter into the slow cooker and cook for 3 hours on low settings. Once done, transfer on a cooling rack and let it cool completely before serving.

Arianna Brooks

Sugar-Free Molten Lava Chocolate Cake

Makes: 1 serving

Carbs per serving: 7.9 grams

Ingredients:

- 1 1/2 cups sweetener (Swerve), divided
- 1/2 cups flour (gluten-free)
- 5 tbsp. cocoa powder, unsweetened, divided
- 1/2 tsp salt
- 1 tsp baking powder
- 1/2 cup butter, melted and cooled
- 3 eggs, whole
- 3 egg yolks
- 1/2 tsp vanilla liquid stevia
- 1 tsp vanilla extract
- 4 oz. chocolate chips (sugar-free)
- 2 cups of hot water

Instructions:

1. Start by greasing the crockpot.
2. Get a large bowl and whisk flour with 3 tbsp. cocoa powder, 1 ¼ cup Swerve, baking powder and salt.
3. In a smaller bowl, stir the whole eggs, egg yolks, liquid stevia, and vanilla extract together with the cooled melted butter.
4. Combine the wet ingredients with the dry ingredients and mix until well combined.
5. Pour the mixture into the crockpot.
6. Put some chocolate chips on top.

7. Combine the remaining 2 tbsp. of cocoa powder and the rest of the sweetener (Swerve) with hot water.
8. Place the cover properly and allow to cook for around 3 hours on low heat setting.
9. Once done, allow the dish to cool slightly. Then serve.

Arianna Brooks

Pumpkin Pie Bars (Sugar-Free)

Makes: 3 servings

Carbs per serving: 6.2 grams

Ingredients:

For the Crust

- 3/4 cup shredded coconut, unsweetened
- 1/4 cup cocoa powder, unsweetened
- 1/2 cup sunflower seed flour or sunflower seeds, raw and unsalted
- 1/4 tsp salt
- 1/4 cup Swerve sweetener
- 4 tbsp. butter, softened

For the Filling

- 6 eggs
- 29 oz. can of pumpkin puree
- 1 cup of heavy cream
- 1 tbsp. pumpkin pie spice
- 1 tbsp. vanilla extract
- 1/2 tsp salt
- 1 tsp pure stevia extract
- 1 tsp cinnamon liquid stevia
- 1/2 cup of sugar-free chocolate chips (optional)

Instructions:

1. Put all the crust ingredients inside a food processor. Process the ingredients until fine crumbs emerge.
2. Grease the bottom of the slow cooker.

3. Evenly press the crust mixture to the bottom. Do it as evenly as you can.
4. Put all the filling ingredients in a blender and process until well combined.
5. If desired, put some chocolate chips on the filling.
6. Pour the mixture on top of the crust.
7. Cover the cooker and allow to cook on low setting for 3 hours.
8. Remove the cover and let the dish cool for half an hour. Refrigerate while still inside the crockpot for a minimum of 3 hours.
9. Slice into small bars and serve.

Arianna Brooks

Dairy and Refined Sugar-Free Fudge

Makes: 1 serving

Carbs per serving: 10.9 grams

Ingredients:

- 2 1/2 cups of chocolate chips, sugar-free
- ¼ cup of raw honey or 2 tsp liquid stevia
- 1/3 cup of coconut milk
- 1 tsp. pure vanilla extract
- 1 pinch of salt

Instructions:

1. Stir together the vanilla, coconut milk, chocolate chips, honey (or stevia) and pinch of salt in a small crockpot (3 or 4-qt. capacity)
2. Cover and let it cook for 2 hours on low heat.
3. Remove the cover, turn the heat of and allow to sit for 1 hour more without stirring.
4. Stir very well for 5 to 10 minutes until consistently smooth.
5. Line a 1-qt casserole dish w/ parchment paper. Pour the mixture.
6. Cover and place inside the refrigerator for 3 to 4 hours or until firm.

Lemon Poke Cake

Makes: 12 servings

Carbs per serving: 7.64 grams

Ingredients:

Cake

- 3 cups of almond flour
- 3/4 cup of sweetener (Swerve)
- 2 tsp baking powder
- 1/4 cup whey protein powder, unflavored
- 4 large-sized eggs (allow to warm at room temperature if refrigerated)
- 1/2 cup cashew or almond milk, unsweetened
- 2 tbsp. lemon juice
- Zest of 1 lemon
- 1 tsp lemon extract
- 1/2 cup of butter, melted
- 1/4 tsp salt
- 1/4 tsp liquid stevia extract

Sugar-Free Lemon Jello:

- 1 cup of boiling water
- 1/4 cup of fresh lemon juice
- 1 tbsp. grass-fed gelatin
- 3 tbsp. Sweetener (Swerve powder)
- 3 drops of yellow veggie-based food coloring (optional, for boosting yellow color only)

Frosting

Arianna Brooks

- 1 cup of whipping cream
- 1/4 cup sweetener (Swerve powder)
- 1/2 tsp of vanilla extract.

Instructions:

Cake

1. Line a 6-qt. slow cooker w/ parchment paper. Make sure there is enough excess parchment on each side to ensure easy removal. Grease the parchment paper.
2. Whisk the almond flour, protein powder, sweetener, salt, and baking powder in a large-sized bowl. Add the eggs, butter, nut milk, lemon extract, lemon juice, lemon zest, and stevia extract and mix until everything is well combined.
3. Prepare the slow cooker and pour batter. Cook on low for about 3 hours. Let it completely cool inside the slow cooker. Get a skewer and poke the cake all over at about half an inch apart. Twist the skewer as you go to create holes.

Jello (prepare while cooling the cake)

1. Mix together the lemon juice and grass-fed gelatin in a small bowl and set aside until the mixture thickens. Put boiling water, yellow food coloring (if desired), sweetener, and gelatin. Stir until the gelatin and sweetener are dissolved completely. Allow to cool until it starts to thicken.

2. Pour the thickened mixture over the cake, allowing the jello to go deep into the cake's holes. Lift the cooker's

ceramic insert and refrigerate for 2 or 3 hours just until the cake sets.
3. Use the excess parchment on the sides to gently lift the cake out. Place it on a serving dish.

Frosting

1. Beat the whipping cream as you add vanilla and sweetener until stiff peaks appear. Spread all over the sides and on top of the cake.

Arianna Brooks

Conclusion

Thank you once again for purchasing this recipe book!

I really hope the recipes in this book were able to help you to create some delicious Low Carb meals that you can make every day with your slow cooker. Now be sure to incorporate these recipes into your cooking to create your healthy meal plan.

Finally, if you enjoyed this book, then I'd like to ask you for a favor, would you be kind enough to leave a review for this book on Amazon? It'd be greatly appreciated! I want to reach as many people as I can with this book and more reviews will help me accomplish that!

You can do that by writing a review in your Amazon account under Your Orders.

Thank you and enjoy!

Printed in Great Britain
by Amazon